The LGBTQ+ Pregnancy and Parenting Guide

Evidence-Based Care from Fertility Through First Year for Transgender, Nonbinary, and Queer Families

Starlet Asasia Murphy

ISBN: 978-1-923646-11-7

First Edition:2025

This book provides educational information about pregnancy, birth, parenting, and family building for LGBTQ+ individuals and families. It is not intended as a substitute for professional medical advice, diagnosis, or treatment. Always seek the advice of qualified healthcare providers regarding medical conditions, treatment options, and health decisions. The authors and publisher disclaim any liability for adverse effects arising from the use or application of information contained in this book.

The case examples throughout this book are fictional composites created for educational purposes. Any resemblance to actual persons, living or deceased, or actual events is purely coincidental. Names, characters, circumstances, and details have been invented to illustrate concepts while protecting privacy. Where real individuals are referenced, they are public figures discussed in appropriate educational context.

Legal information provided is general in nature and may not reflect current law in all jurisdictions. Laws regarding parental rights, adoption, birth certificates, and LGBTQ+ family recognition vary significantly by state and country and change frequently. Readers must consult qualified attorneys in their jurisdiction for legal advice specific to their circumstances. The authors and publisher are not responsible for legal outcomes resulting from information in this book.

Medical information reflects current research and clinical guidelines as of publication date but medical knowledge evolves rapidly. Treatment recommendations, medication safety information, and clinical protocols may change. Readers should verify current medical guidelines with healthcare providers before making medical decisions. The authors and publisher are not liable for medical outcomes.

Financial information about fertility treatments, surrogacy, and family building costs are estimates based on current market rates and may vary significantly by location and provider. Readers should verify costs directly with providers and financial advisors before making financial commitments.

Product recommendations, resource listings, and organizational references are provided for informational purposes only and do not constitute endorsements. The authors and publisher have no financial relationships with listed organizations unless explicitly stated. Inclusion or exclusion of resources does not imply quality judgment.

This book discusses sensitive topics including pregnancy loss, discrimination, mental health challenges, and medical procedures. Some content may be emotionally difficult. Readers experiencing crisis should contact appropriate emergency services or crisis support resources immediately rather than relying solely on this book.

By reading this book, you acknowledge that you understand and accept these limitations and disclaimers. The information provided is offered in good faith to support LGBTQ+ families, but individual circumstances vary and professional guidance tailored to your specific situation is essential.

Table of Contents

Introduction

When Elena and her wife Jasmine walked into their first prenatal appointment, the intake form asked which one was the "mother" and which was the "father." The nurse looked confused when Elena explained they were both mothers. The obstetrician referred to Elena's body parts with language that felt clinical and disconnected. Nobody seemed to understand that Jasmine carried equal importance in this pregnancy journey, even though Elena's body was doing the growing.

When Marcus, a transgender man, confirmed his pregnancy, his family doctor congratulated him and then admitted she had no idea how to provide appropriate care. Should he stop testosterone? When? How would pregnancy affect his transition? Could he chest-feed after top surgery? The doctor meant well but had no framework for understanding his experience.

When David and his husband Carlos began exploring surrogacy, they found countless resources about the IVF process and legal contracts, but almost nothing about the emotional journey of becoming parents through another person's pregnancy, or how to build connection with their baby when they couldn't feel those kicks themselves.

These aren't unusual stories. They're the norm.

The Gap That Shouldn't Exist

Here's the reality: LGBTQ+ people have been having babies forever. We've been creating families, carrying pregnancies, supporting partners, and birthing children since the beginning of human history. What's changed isn't our existence—it's our visibility and our increasing unwillingness to accept healthcare that erases us.

Yet when you search for comprehensive pregnancy resources that actually speak to LGBTQ+ experiences, you'll find a startling gap. A few books cover conception and fertility—how to get pregnant when your relationship doesn't include the right combination of reproductive parts. That's helpful, but it's just the beginning. Once you're pregnant, the resources essentially disappear. You're left cobbling together information from mainstream pregnancy books written with exclusively heterosexual, cisgender audiences in mind, translating language that doesn't fit, and navigating systems that weren't designed with you in consideration.

The American College of Nurse-Midwives now explicitly includes LGBTQ+ cultural competency in their core competencies for practice (American College of Nurse-Midwives, 2020). Certification exams test on inclusive care. Professional standards demand it. But where's the actual resource that brings this knowledge together? Where's the comprehensive guide that takes LGBTQ+ families from conception through postpartum with affirming, evidence-based, practical information?

That's why this book exists.

Who This Book Is For

This book is for you if you're:

A lesbian or queer woman planning pregnancy with your partner, navigating sperm donor decisions, or already pregnant and wanting care that honors your relationship and family structure.

A transgender man considering pregnancy, managing the complex intersection of your gender identity and reproductive capacity, or needing guidance on stopping testosterone, navigating pregnancy in a male body, or chest-feeding after top surgery.

A non-binary person who's pregnant or planning pregnancy, needing language and frameworks that honor your identity while accessing care in gendered systems.

A gay male couple pursuing surrogacy and wanting more than just legal and medical logistics—seeking to understand how to become parents when someone else carries your child.

A queer-identified person of any gender whose family doesn't fit conventional categories, who needs care providers to understand your chosen family structure, your language preferences, and your unique path to parenthood.

A single LGBTQ+ parent by choice, creating your family intentionally outside of partnership, needing resources that don't assume a co-parent exists.

Part of a polyamorous family where multiple people share parenting roles and responsibilities, navigating systems that only recognize two parents.

An LGBTQ+ person using assisted reproductive technology and needing guidance that goes beyond the mechanics of IVF or IUI to address your specific questions and concerns.

This book is also for healthcare providers—midwives, obstetricians, nurses, doulas, and other birth workers—who want to provide truly affirming care and need comprehensive guidance on the specific considerations for LGBTQ+ pregnancies and families.

How to Use This Guide

This isn't a book you necessarily read straight through from beginning to end (though you certainly can). It's designed to meet you wherever you are in your journey.

If you're just starting to think about having a baby, begin with Part One: Foundations (Chapters 1.0-4.0). These chapters help you understand your options, plan your family, choose your care team, and understand your body's fertility.

If you're actively trying to conceive, jump to Part Two: Conception Pathways (Chapters 5.0-9.0). Find the chapter that matches your family configuration and conception method. These chapters provide specific, practical guidance for your situation.

If you're already pregnant, head to Part Three: Pregnancy Journey (Chapters 10.0-15.0). These chapters guide you through each trimester with attention to LGBTQ+ specific considerations alongside standard prenatal care information.

If you're preparing for birth, Part Four: Birth Preparation and Labor (Chapters 16.0-20.0) walks you through creating your birth plan, preparing your hospital or birth center, understanding labor and birth, and addressing special considerations.

If you've given birth and are in the postpartum period, Part Five: Postpartum and Feeding (Chapters 21.0-26.0) addresses recovery, feeding options, mental health, and newborn care with LGBTQ+ families in mind.

If you're dealing with specific challenges, Part Six: Special Topics and Advocacy (Chapters 27.0-30.0) covers high-risk pregnancy, pregnancy loss, legal rights, and advocacy strategies.

Throughout the book, you'll find:

Real Stories from diverse LGBTQ+ families (with names changed and identifying details modified to protect privacy). These aren't my stories—they're composite examples drawn from patterns I've witnessed in practice and research, representing the breadth of experiences in our community.

Midwife's Perspective boxes that provide clinical insights and evidence-based guidance on specific topics.

Partner Spotlight sections offering information specifically for non-gestational partners, because your role matters enormously.

Affirmation Boxes for moments when you need validation that your feelings, questions, or experiences are completely normal and reasonable.

Red Flag/Green Flag guidance to help you identify affirming versus problematic care.

Evidence Summary sections highlighting key research findings with full citations, because you deserve to know that information is backed by actual science.

Reflection Questions embedded throughout to help you process what you're reading and apply it to your situation.

Action Steps providing concrete next steps you can take right now.

Resource Boxes pointing you to specific tools, websites, organizations, and support networks.

A Note on Language and Inclusivity

Language matters. It matters a lot when we're talking about bodies, identities, families, and one of the most vulnerable experiences humans go through.

Throughout this book, I've made specific choices about language, and I want to be transparent about those choices:

Anatomical terms: I use both medical terminology and more inclusive language. You'll see "pregnant person" alongside "pregnant woman" depending on context. I use "chest-feeding" and "breastfeeding" interchangeably because different people prefer different terms. I refer to "gestational parent" and "non-gestational parent" when needed, but also "mother," "father," and "parent" as appropriate. When discussing anatomy, I sometimes use clinical terms (uterus, cervix, testes) and sometimes more colloquial language, always with the goal of clarity.

Gender and identity: I use people's self-identified terms. A transgender man who becomes pregnant is still a man. A non-binary person is neither male nor female, regardless of their anatomy or reproductive capacity. Lesbian and queer women are women. Gender identity and reproductive capacity are separate things that sometimes overlap in complicated ways.

Family structures: I don't assume family composition. Partners might be spouses or not, married or not, the same gender or not, two people or more than two. Some people parent alone by choice. Some involve close friends or chosen family. I try to use language that encompasses all these possibilities.

Pronouns: I alternate between he, she, and they throughout the book in examples and general references, reflecting the diversity of people who might be pregnant or parenting. In specific examples, I use the pronouns appropriate to that person's identity.

What I won't do: I won't use language that erases identity. I won't call a transgender man a woman just because he's pregnant. I won't refer to a non-gestational mother as a father. I won't use scare quotes around people's identities or chosen terminology. I won't prioritize medical convenience over human dignity.

What I ask of you: Use whatever language feels right for your body and your identity. When I use a term that doesn't fit you, mentally substitute the one that does. If you're a trans man who prefers "breastfeeding" to "chest-feeding," use it. If you're a cisgender lesbian who dislikes "birthing person" and prefers "pregnant woman," claim it. This book provides options, not prescriptions.

The language in this book reflects 2024-2025 conventions in LGBTQ+ communities and healthcare. Language evolves, and what feels affirming now might shift. The principle remains constant: people get to define themselves, and healthcare should adapt to people—not the other way around.

Meet the Author and Acknowledgment of Community Expertise

A note on authorship and expertise: While this book is written from a midwifery perspective and draws on extensive clinical experience, it's been informed by something far more important—the lived experiences of LGBTQ+ people who've navigated pregnancy and birth in systems that weren't designed for them.

No single person can represent the full diversity of LGBTQ+ family experiences. A cisgender lesbian couple's journey differs substantially from a transgender man's pregnancy experience, which differs from gay male couple's surrogacy path, which differs from a non-binary person's birth story. Each deserves attention, respect, and specific guidance.

This book synthesizes current research on LGBTQ+ reproductive health (which has grown substantially in recent years but remains insufficient), clinical guidelines from organizations like the American College of Nurse-Midwives and the American College of Obstetricians and Gynecologists, published first-person accounts from LGBTQ+ parents, and practice wisdom from providers who've dedicated themselves to affirming care.

Where research exists, it's cited. Where gaps exist (and there are many), the book acknowledges uncertainty while providing the best available guidance based on clinical experience and related research. The field of LGBTQ+ perinatal health is young. We're building the evidence base as we go, and LGBTQ+ families are leading the way.

This book stands on the shoulders of activists, clinicians, researchers, and LGBTQ+ parents who've fought for visibility, demanded better care, shared their stories, and refused to accept erasure. It owes a debt to the couples who educate their providers, the transgender men who've navigated pregnancy with grace despite inadequate support, the lesbian mothers who've advocated for their family recognition, the gay fathers who've built families through surrogacy and adoption, and the non-binary people who've insisted that gender and reproduction are more complex than binary systems acknowledge.

To everyone whose experience helped shape this resource: thank you. Your courage in creating families despite systemic barriers has paved the way for better care, more research, and increased visibility. This book exists because of you.

Now let's get to the practical guidance you came here for.

Starlet Asasia Murphy

Chapter Overview and Pathways for Different Readers

This book contains 30 chapters organized into six parts, moving chronologically through the journey from conception planning through postpartum. Here's the roadmap:

Part One: Foundations (Chapters 1.0-4.0)

These chapters establish the groundwork everyone needs, regardless of family configuration or conception method. Chapter 1.0 addresses language, identity, and self-advocacy. Chapter 2.0 covers family planning specific to LGBTQ+ people. Chapter 3.0 guides you through choosing affirming care providers. Chapter 4.0 explains fertility and reproductive anatomy across different body types and identities.

Start here if: You're just beginning to consider pregnancy, want to understand your options, or need to build your knowledge foundation before diving into specifics.

Part Two: Conception Pathways (Chapters 5.0-9.0)

These chapters provide detailed guidance for different family configurations and conception methods. Chapter 5.0 addresses conception for lesbian and queer couples. Chapter 6.0 focuses on transgender men and non-binary people. Chapter 7.0 covers surrogacy for gay male couples. Chapter 8.0 discusses alternative family configurations including polyamory and co-parenting. Chapter 9.0 addresses fertility challenges and when conception takes longer than expected.

Start here if: You're actively trying to conceive or have a clear plan for your conception method and want specific guidance for your situation.

Part Three: Pregnancy Journey (Chapters 10.0-15.0)

These chapters walk through pregnancy trimester by trimester, with specific attention to LGBTQ+ experiences. Chapters 10.0-12.0 cover first, second, and third trimesters. Chapter 13.0 provides detailed guidance for trans and non-binary pregnant people. Chapter 14.0 focuses on partner involvement and co-parenting during pregnancy. Chapter 15.0 addresses prenatal mental health and identity.

Start here if: You're already pregnant and want guidance on prenatal care, physical changes, and preparing for birth while navigating your identity and relationships.

Part Four: Birth Preparation and Labor (Chapters 16.0-20.0)

These chapters prepare you for labor and birth. Chapter 16.0 guides you through creating inclusive birth preferences. Chapter 17.0 addresses preparing hospitals and birth centers for your needs. Chapters 18.0-19.0 explain labor, birth, and medical interventions from a midwifery perspective. Chapter 20.0 provides special guidance for trans and non-binary people during birth.

Start here if: You're in your third trimester, planning your birth, or want to understand what happens during labor and delivery with attention to LGBTQ+ considerations.

Part Five: Postpartum and Feeding (Chapters 21.0-26.0)

These chapters address the immediate postpartum period and beyond. Chapters 21.0-22.0 cover the first hours and first six weeks after birth. Chapters 23.0-24.0 provide comprehensive guidance on feeding options including chest-feeding, induced lactation, and formula feeding. Chapters 25.0-26.0 address postpartum mental health and newborn care as LGBTQ+ parents.

Start here if: You've given birth, are preparing for postpartum, or specifically need guidance on feeding options or recovery.

Part Six: Special Topics and Advocacy (Chapters 27.0-30.0)

These chapters address specific challenges and advocacy needs. Chapter 27.0 covers high-risk pregnancy considerations. Chapter 28.0 addresses pregnancy loss and grief. Chapter 29.0 explains legal rights and documentation. Chapter 30.0 provides advocacy strategies and guides you in creating systemic change.

Start here if: You're dealing with medical complications, pregnancy loss, legal challenges, or want to advocate for better care within systems.

Quick Reference Guide by Family Type

For Lesbian and Queer Female Couples

Essential chapters: 1.0, 2.0, 3.0, 4.0, 5.0, then 10.0-15.0, 16.0-19.0, 21.0-26.0

Skip if desired: 6.0 (trans-specific conception), 7.0 (surrogacy), 13.0 (trans-specific pregnancy), 20.0 (trans-specific birth)

Consider: 9.0 if conception takes time, 14.0 for partner involvement, 23.0-24.0 for feeding including induced lactation

For Transgender Men

Essential chapters: 1.0, 2.0, 3.0, 4.0, 6.0, then 10.0, 11.0, 12.0, 13.0, 15.0, 16.0, 17.0, 18.0, 19.0, 20.0, 21.0-26.0

Skip if desired: 5.0 (lesbian-specific conception), 7.0 (surrogacy)

Consider: 9.0 if conception challenges arise, 14.0 if partnered, 25.0 for mental health support, 24.0 for chest-feeding options

For Non-Binary Pregnant People

Essential chapters: 1.0, 2.0, 3.0, 4.0, then 10.0, 11.0, 12.0, 13.0, 15.0, 16.0, 17.0, 18.0, 19.0, 20.0, 21.0-26.0

Consider: 5.0 or 6.0 depending on conception method, 9.0 if fertility challenges, 14.0 if partnered, 25.0 for mental health

For Gay Male Couples Using Surrogacy

Essential chapters: 1.0, 2.0, 3.0, 7.0, 14.0, 21.0, 22.0, 23.0, 26.0

Consider: 4.0 for understanding fertility and IVF process, 9.0 if facing conception challenges, 25.0 for postpartum mental health, 27.0 if complications arise

For Single LGBTQ+ Parents

Essential chapters: 1.0, 2.0, 3.0, 4.0, 8.0, then pregnancy/birth/postpartum chapters based on your body and situation

Skip: 14.0 (partner-focused), though some guidance on support networks still applies

For Polyamorous or Co-Parenting Families

Essential chapters: 1.0, 2.0, 3.0, 8.0, then chapters based on who's carrying and conception method, plus 29.0 for legal considerations

Consider: All pregnancy/birth/postpartum chapters based on gestational parent's body and needs, 14.0 adapted for multiple partners

For Healthcare Providers

Essential reading: All of Part One (1.0-4.0), Chapter 13.0 (trans pregnancy), Chapter 17.0 (preparing facilities), Chapter 20.0 (trans birth), Chapter 29.0 (legal rights), Chapter 30.0 (advocacy)

Recommended: Sample chapters from Parts 2, 3, 4, and 5 to understand patient experiences and concerns across different family types

Emergency Resources and Hotlines

Keep these resources accessible throughout your pregnancy journey:

Crisis Support

The Trevor Project (LGBTQ+ youth crisis support, but serves young adults too)

- Phone: 1-866-488-7386
- Text: Text START to 678-678
- Available 24/7

Trans Lifeline (peer support by and for trans people)

- US: 1-877-565-8860
- Canada: 1-877-330-6366
- Available varies by volunteer availability

National Suicide Prevention Lifeline

- Phone: 988
- Available 24/7
- Now includes specific training on LGBTQ+ issues

Postpartum Support International (for perinatal mental health crises)

- Phone: 1-800-944-4773
- Text: 800-944-4773
- Available 24/7 hotline, business hours for text

Medical Emergency

Always call 911 for medical emergencies. Concerns about provider discrimination should never prevent you from seeking emergency care.

Pregnancy-related reasons to seek immediate emergency care:

- Severe abdominal pain
- Heavy bleeding (soaking through a pad in an hour or less)
- Severe headache with visual changes or swelling
- Reduced or absent fetal movement after 28 weeks
- Fluid leaking from vagina before 37 weeks
- Signs of preterm labor before 37 weeks
- Thoughts of harming yourself or your baby

Legal and Advocacy Support

Lambda Legal (LGBTQ+ legal support and discrimination cases)

- Help Desk: 1-866-542-8336
- www.lambdalegal.org

National Center for Lesbian Rights

- Phone: 1-800-528-6257
- www.nclrights.org
- Provides legal information and referrals

GLBTQ Legal Advocates & Defenders (GLAD)

- Phone: 1-800-455-4523
- www.glad.org
- Answers Legal InfoLine calls and provides resources

Healthcare Navigation

LGBTQ+ Healthcare Provider Directories:

- GLMA (Gay and Lesbian Medical Association): www.glma.org/provider-directory
- World Professional Association for Transgender Health: www.wpath.org/provider/search

- Refuge Restrooms (for finding safe, accessible bathrooms): www.refugerestrooms.org

Community Support

Family Equality (support and advocacy for LGBTQ+ families)

- www.familyequality.org
- Connects families with local resources and support groups

Colage (for people with LGBTQ+ parents, but offers community connection)

- www.colage.org

Online Communities:

- LGBTQ+ pregnancy and parenting groups on Facebook (search for specific groups for your identity/situation)
- Reddit communities: r/queerception, r/lgbtparenting
- Local LGBTQ+ parenting groups (search in your area)

Book-Specific Resources

This book includes extensive resources at the end of each chapter and in the appendices. Appendix C provides a comprehensive directory of LGBTQ+ birth professionals by region. Appendix A includes detailed question banks for interviewing providers. Appendix B offers document templates for birth preferences, hospital communication, and legal agreements.

Part One: Foundations

Chapter 1.0: Language Identity and Pregnancy

When Jordan scheduled their first prenatal appointment, the receptionist paused. "So... are you the mother?" Jordan took a breath. "I'm pregnant, yes. I use they/them pronouns." Another pause. "Okay, but for the medical records, we need to know if you're the mother or the father." Jordan felt that familiar tightness in their chest—the one that comes when you have to choose between being seen and being heard.

This wasn't Jordan's first rodeo with healthcare systems that couldn't quite figure out what to do with people who don't fit neat boxes. But pregnancy? This was different. This was months of appointments, strangers touching their body, forms that didn't make sense, and language that felt wrong in ways that were hard to articulate.

Language shapes how we experience the world, and nowhere is this truer than in pregnancy and birth. The words used to describe your body, your family, your experience—they matter. They can make you feel seen or erased, respected or dismissed, human or clinical. And here's the thing about pregnancy in LGBTQ+ communities: we've been doing this forever, but the language hasn't caught up.

1.1 Why Words Matter Now

Pregnancy makes you vulnerable in ways you might not expect. Your body changes. You need medical care. You interact with systems—hospitals, insurance companies, legal institutions—that have power over you and your growing family. In these moments, language isn't just about being polite. It's about dignity, safety, and whether you can trust the people taking care of you.

Research confirms what LGBTQ+ people already know: experiences of discrimination in healthcare settings directly impact health outcomes (Lamda Legal, 2010). When transgender men report avoiding prenatal care due to fear of mistreatment, that's not oversensitivity—that's a rational response to documented patterns of discrimination (Hoffkling et al., 2017). When lesbian couples describe feeling invisible during pregnancy, with providers directing all conversation to the gestational parent while ignoring the partner, that erasure has real consequences for family bonding and postpartum mental health (Ross et al., 2006).

The words matter because they signal safety. They tell you if this provider gets it, if this space is for you too, if you can relax into care or if you need to stay guarded and ready to educate or defend.

1.2 The Terminology Landscape

Let's get oriented to the language you'll encounter and the choices you'll need to make about what fits for you.

Pregnant person vs. pregnant woman: Many inclusive spaces now use "pregnant person" to acknowledge that not everyone who can become pregnant identifies as a woman. Transgender men can become pregnant. Non-binary people can become pregnant. But many cisgender women find "pregnant person" alienating or depersonalizing. There's no single right answer. Use what fits your identity, and expect good providers to ask what you prefer rather than assuming.

Birthing person vs. mother: Similar logic applies here. "Mother" carries profound meaning for many people and erasing it feels wrong. But for transgender men who give birth, being called "mother" can feel deeply incorrect—they're fathers, or parents, but not mothers. Some non-binary people claim "mother," others use "parent" or invent new terms entirely. You get to choose.

Chest-feeding vs. breastfeeding: This one generates surprising amounts of controversy. "Chest-feeding" emerged from transgender and non-binary communities to describe feeding a baby from one's chest without the gendered language of "breast." Some people love it. Some transgender men prefer "breastfeeding" because it's medically accurate and they're not bothered by the term. Some non-binary people use them interchangeably. All of these choices are valid.

Partner vs. spouse vs. co-parent vs. other terms: The language for non-gestational parents in LGBTQ+ families varies widely. "Partner" is common but doesn't capture legal relationships. "Spouse" works if you're married but excludes non-married partners. "Co-parent" is neutral but can feel clinical. Some families invent their own terms. What matters is that your care team uses the language you specify.

Anatomy terms: Here's where things get tricky. Medical language for reproductive anatomy is gendered—vagina, cervix, uterus, breasts. Some transgender men and non-binary people prefer gender-neutral terms like "front hole" or "chest" or "lower anatomy." Others use standard medical terms without issue because they separate body parts from gender identity. Providers should ask what language you want used when discussing your body, then use that language consistently (Obedin-Maliver & Makadon, 2016).

Think about what language feels right for your body and your identity. Nobody can tell you what words should fit. Some transgender men are fine with clinical terms for anatomy while insisting on male pronouns and being called "father." Some non-binary people want entirely gender-neutral language across the board. Some lesbian mothers want specifically feminine language that acknowledges the female body. You're the expert on your own experience.

1.3 Documentation and Medical Records

Here's a reality check: medical systems were designed with cisgender, heterosexual people in mind, and the documentation reflects that. Electronic medical records have fields for "mother" and "father," sometimes "parent 1" and "parent 2," rarely space for three or more parents. Gender fields often offer only male/female, maybe "other" if you're lucky. Pregnancy templates assume the pregnant person uses she/her pronouns.

You'll encounter forms that don't work for you. Guaranteed. The question isn't if but how you'll handle it.

Name and pronoun documentation: Most healthcare systems now include fields for "name used" and "legal name," plus pronouns. If your provider's system has these fields, use them. If not, write your name and pronouns prominently on every form. Some people put pronouns in the top corner: "They/Them" or "He/Him" or whatever applies. Some write notes in margins: "I'm transgender—please use male pronouns." Some verbally correct staff every time. All valid strategies.

The Americans with Disabilities Act and various state laws increasingly protect the right to be addressed by your correct name and pronouns in healthcare settings (National Center for Transgender Equality, 2021). If staff persistently use wrong names or pronouns after being corrected, that's not just rudeness—it may be discrimination you can formally address.

Gender markers: If your legal gender marker doesn't match your identity or reproductive capacity, you'll navigate confusing systems. Insurance companies sometimes deny coverage for "gender-inappropriate" services—like denying pregnancy-related care for someone with a male gender marker. You may need your provider to code services carefully or write letters of medical necessity. Some people change legal gender markers before pregnancy. Others handle the paperwork complications. Neither choice is wrong.

Partner documentation: If you have a non-gestational partner who will be actively involved in your care and birth, get their name in your chart early. Some systems have "support person" or "emergency contact" fields that can establish their legitimacy. If you're married, that helps legally. If you're not married or if you have multiple partners, the documentation gets trickier, but starting early helps.

1.4 Navigating Provider Interactions

You'll work with multiple providers throughout pregnancy: midwives or obstetricians, nurses, ultrasound technicians, lab staff, possibly specialists. Each interaction is a chance to set the tone.

First appointments set precedent: When you first meet a provider, establish your language preferences clearly. "I'm pregnant and I use he/him pronouns. I prefer to be called a father, not a mother. I'd like you to refer to my anatomy using standard medical terms—that works fine for me." Or: "I'm non-binary and I use they/them pronouns. I'd appreciate if you use gender-neutral language throughout—'pregnant person' rather than 'pregnant woman,' and 'chest' rather than 'breasts.'"

Most providers appreciate direct guidance. They want to get it right but don't always know what you need unless you tell them. Think of this first conversation as training—you're teaching them how to care for you specifically.

Handling mistakes gracefully (when you can): Staff will mess up your pronouns. They'll use the wrong words. This happens even with the most affirming providers because humans are imperfect and healthcare workers are busy and distracted. You get to decide how much energy you put into corrections.

Some people correct every mistake: "He, not she." Others let small mistakes slide and only address patterns. Some have partners do the correcting to reduce their own labor. Figure out what's sustainable for you. You're not obligated to educate people or be patient with repeated mistakes, especially if you've already provided clear guidance.

When to escalate: If a provider or staff member is actively disrespectful—using wrong pronouns after multiple corrections, making comments about your family structure, expressing personal discomfort with your identity—don't tough it out. Talk to the practice manager or switch providers. Discrimination is not okay, even if it's subtle or couched as personal beliefs.

Consider this situation (a composite I've observed): Marcus, a transgender man in his second trimester, worked with a midwife who seemed fine initially. But she kept "forgetting" his pronouns, calling him "mama" despite his repeated corrections, and making comments like "Well, you're doing something only women can do." Marcus initially tried to be patient, thinking she'd adjust. But by week 20, his stress around appointments was affecting his mental health. He switched to a different practice and immediately felt the difference. The new midwife got his pronouns right consistently, never made assumptions, and treated his pregnancy as exactly what it was—a man having a baby.

You don't owe anyone patience if they're not trying. Your mental health and sense of safety matter more than being nice to providers who won't respect you.

1.5 Self Advocacy Strategies

Self-advocacy means speaking up for your needs, even when it's uncomfortable. Pregnancy amplifies this need because you're more vulnerable and more dependent on systems.

Prepare talking points: Before appointments, think through what you need to communicate. Write it down if that helps. Examples: "I need you to use they/them pronouns," "My partner will be at all appointments and should receive all information," "I prefer 'chest-feeding' to 'breastfeeding,'" "I want my legal name on billing but my chosen name everywhere else."

Bring backup: Partners, friends, doulas—whoever can support you. They can help correct pronouns, take notes, ask questions you forget, and advocate for you when you're tired or stressed. Non-gestational partners often become expert advocates because they're not the one being examined and can focus on communication.

Document everything: Keep notes on who said what, especially if there are problems. Write down names of staff members who are great and ones who are problematic. This documentation helps if you need to file complaints or if you're trying to ensure you work with specific people.

Know your rights: You have rights to respectful care, to decline procedures, to have support people present (within reason—COVID changed some of these norms), to informed consent, and to file complaints about discrimination. The National Center for Transgender Equality and Lambda Legal provide state-by-state guides to legal protections (Lambda Legal, 2020).

Practice assertiveness: If you're not naturally assertive, this skill matters in pregnancy. Practice phrases: "That doesn't work for me," "I need you to use different language," "Stop and explain this to me," "I'd like to think about that before deciding." You're allowed to be direct about your needs.

1.6 When Standard Language Fails

Sometimes medical language just doesn't fit your experience, and you need to create your own vocabulary.

Elena and Jasmine (a lesbian couple) faced this when Elena was pregnant with their first child. Medical forms and providers kept treating Jasmine as a support person rather than a parent. They started using "co-mother" and "gestational mother" to clarify both their roles. Elena was the gestational mother—her body was pregnant. Jasmine was the non-gestational mother—equally a parent from conception. This language helped providers understand that both needed information, both were making decisions, and both were parents from day one.

River, a non-binary person, found that neither "mother" nor "father" fit. They eventually settled on "ren"—a shortened version of "parent" that felt more personal than the full word but didn't carry gendered weight. Their care team picked it up quickly: "How is ren feeling today?" "Ren's blood pressure looks good." The language wasn't standard medical terminology, but it honored River's identity while communicating clearly.

Some transgender men reclaim female anatomy words, using "my vagina" and "my uterus" because those are their body parts and they're comfortable with clinical language. Others create elaborate workarounds to avoid gendered terms. Neither approach is more valid. What matters is that your language reflects your truth.

If you're creating new vocabulary, bring your care team in early. Explain what words you're using and why. Most providers adapt readily if you give clear guidance. The ones who can't adapt might not be the right fit for you.

1.7 Building Your Vocabulary Toolkit

Affirmation Boxes: You're Not Being Difficult

Asking for language that fits your identity isn't demanding special treatment. It's requiring basic respect. Healthcare is supposed to be patient-centered. That means centering your actual identity, not the one providers assume based on your anatomy.

Reflection Questions

What words for your body feel most comfortable? Which ones make you cringe?

How important is it that partners or support people share your language preferences versus using their own terms?

What's your threshold for educating providers versus simply requiring correct language?

Creating Your Personal Glossary

Make a list of terms you want your care team to use:

- Your pronouns
- Terms for your role (mother, father, parent, ren, other)
- Terms for your anatomy (standard medical terms, gender-neutral alternatives, or something else)
- Terms for your partner's role
- Terms for conception method (donor, known donor, reciprocal IVF, etc.)
- Terms for feeding plan (chest-feeding, breastfeeding, formula feeding, etc.)

Share this list at your first appointment. Some people even create a one-page document to include in their chart that explains their identity, family structure, and language preferences. It saves repeated explanations and ensures everyone on the care team has the information.

1.8 Moving Forward With Clarity

Language is the foundation of how you'll experience pregnancy care. Getting this right early makes everything else easier. You shouldn't have to repeatedly correct providers or feel misunderstood at every appointment. You deserve care that sees you clearly.

As you move into family planning (which we'll cover in Chapter 2.0), choosing your care team (Chapter 3.0), and understanding your fertility (Chapter 4.0), you'll apply these language principles throughout. Every interaction, every decision, every question you ask will be filtered through how comfortable you feel with the words being used.

Start now with clarifying your own vocabulary. What words feel right? What makes you cringe? Which providers honor your language and which ones resist? These answers guide you toward affirming care and away from situations where you'll need to be constantly defensive.

You're growing a baby and building a family. The language used to describe that reality should honor both the biology and the identity. Anything less isn't good enough.

Chapter 2.0: Family Planning for LGBTQ People

Most pregnancy books start with "deciding if you're ready to have a baby." This one starts different: you've already decided. The question isn't if but how, and that "how" gets complicated fast when you're LGBTQ+.

Straight couples who can accidentally get pregnant have the luxury of not planning every single detail. They can decide they want a baby and see what happens. LGBTQ+ family building requires intention. Logistics. Money. Legal protections. Sometimes medical intervention. Sometimes multiple people's bodies and decisions coordinating. The planning phase isn't optional—it's the necessary groundwork that determines if and how your family happens.

This chapter covers the practical and financial realities of LGBTQ+ family planning: defining what you actually want your family to look like, timing considerations unique to queer families, the financial planning required, insurance navigation, legal protections, and fertility preservation options. Think of this as the strategic planning session before the action begins.

2.1 Defining Your Family Vision

Before you start researching fertility clinics or interviewing midwives, get clear on what you actually want. LGBTQ+ family formation offers options that don't exist in straight paradigms, but options create complexity.

Who will be parents? Seems obvious until you're in a polyamorous relationship or a co-parenting arrangement. Some families have two parents. Some have three or four. Some have one parent plus a known donor who remains involved. Some include close friends or chosen family as additional caregivers without legal parent status. Define early who's in and what roles people play.

Who will carry the pregnancy (if applicable)? In lesbian couples, this decision involves biology, career timing, health factors, and sometimes deep emotional considerations about who wants the pregnancy experience. Some couples know immediately. Others agonize. Some do reciprocal IVF so both partners contribute biologically. Some switch who carries for different children.

Research on lesbian couples shows that the decision of who carries often reflects complex negotiations around biological connection, career demands, age-related fertility, and deeply held desires about experiencing pregnancy (Chabot & Ames, 2004). There's no right answer, just the answer that fits your relationship and circumstances.

What does biological connection mean to you? LGBTQ+ families navigate this differently than straight families. In lesbian couples, one partner might carry using the other partner's eggs (reciprocal IVF), creating biological connection for both. In gay male couples using surrogacy, usually one partner provides sperm, but some mix sperm to leave biological parentage uncertain. In transgender families, the pregnant person's biology is clear but how that factors into parent roles varies.

Get honest about how much biological connection matters to you. Some people care deeply. Others care not at all. Some discover feelings changing as they go through the process. No judgment—just clarity about what you're working with.

How do you envision birth and early parenting? Who attends the birth? Who does middle-of-the-night feedings? If there's a gestational parent and a non-gestational parent, how do you ensure both bond with the baby? If there are more than two parents, how do you divide responsibilities and time?

Lesbian couples who plan for equitable parenting from the start report better relationship satisfaction and less postpartum distress

(Goldberg & Perry-Jenkins, 2007). Thinking through these questions before pregnancy helps avoid assumptions and resentments.

2.2 Timing Considerations

Straight couples can simply "try" until pregnancy happens. LGBTQ+ family building involves coordination and resources that make timing decisions more complex.

Biological age and fertility windows: If you're using eggs or sperm that will decline with age, that's a factor. Female fertility declines significantly after 35. If a lesbian couple is deciding who carries, age might influence the choice. If a transgender man stops testosterone to become pregnant, timing affects how long he's off hormones. If gay male couples are using egg donors, younger donors have higher success rates but cost more.

Financial readiness: Conception for LGBTQ+ families usually costs money upfront—sperm banks, fertility treatments, legal fees, surrogacy costs. Unlike straight couples who can time conception around their sexual activity, you're often timing it around when you can afford the next round of treatment. We'll cover finances in section 2.3, but recognize that money constraints affect timing decisions.

Career and life circumstances: Pregnancy and early parenting affect careers. Who can afford time off? Who has parental leave? Who has health insurance that covers maternity care? If you're a graduate student, timing around academic milestones matters. If you're in a demanding job, timing around promotion cycles matters. If you're transitioning medically, timing around those treatments matters.

Relationship stability: If you're partnered, relationship stability matters. Some people jump into pregnancy early in relationships because biological clocks are ticking. Others wait for established stability. Neither choice is wrong, but LGBTQ+ relationship recognition laws vary by state, affecting legal protections if relationships end.

Legal landscape: State laws about parental recognition change. Some LGBTQ+ families time conception around moving to more supportive states or jurisdictions. Some wait for legal marriage if that secures parental rights. Some proceed knowing they'll fight legal battles if needed. Understanding your state's laws helps time decisions strategically.

2.3 Financial Planning

Let's talk money honestly. LGBTQ+ family building often requires financial resources that straight couples don't need.

Conception costs: Home insemination using known donor sperm costs minimal money (equipment, storage, timing). Unknown donor sperm from sperm banks costs $500-$1,000 per vial plus shipping. Intrauterine insemination (IUI) at fertility clinics costs $300-$1,000 per cycle plus sperm costs. In vitro fertilization (IVF) costs $12,000-$25,000 per cycle depending on location and clinic (American Society for Reproductive Medicine, 2023). Surrogacy costs $100,000-$150,000+ including agency fees, medical costs, and surrogate compensation.

Most lesbian couples pursuing pregnancy will spend $2,000-$10,000 if it works within a few cycles of IUI. If IVF becomes necessary, costs escalate. Gay male couples using surrogacy face six-figure expenses from the start. Transgender men may or may not need fertility treatments depending on their conception approach.

Medical costs: Prenatal care, birth, and postpartum care cost money even with insurance. Hospital births in the US average $10,000-$15,000 before insurance (March of Dimes, 2021). Birth center births cost $3,000-$6,000. Home births cost $3,000-$5,000. Your insurance coverage determines out-of-pocket expenses.

Legal costs: Second-parent adoption costs $1,500-$5,000 depending on state and whether you use an attorney. Donor agreements with known donors cost $500-$1,500 for legal drafting. Surrogacy agreements cost significantly more. Pre-birth orders establishing parental rights cost $3,000-$8,000 in states where they're available.

Fertility preservation: If you're a transgender person considering medical transition, fertility preservation before hormones or surgery costs money. Egg freezing costs $8,000-$15,000 plus annual storage fees. Sperm banking costs $1,000-$2,000 initially plus storage.

Time off work: Pregnancy, birth, and early parenting involve time away from work. Parental leave policies vary widely. Some people have paid leave. Many don't. Calculate income loss alongside direct expenses.

Add it all up. The total cost of LGBTQ+ family building from conception through the first year varies from $5,000 on the low end (using known donor, straightforward pregnancy, supportive employer, good insurance) to $200,000+ on the high end (surrogacy or extensive fertility treatments, legal battles, no paid leave, poor insurance).

Plan realistically. Save money if possible. Consider grants and programs specifically for LGBTQ+ family building—organizations like Family Equality offer some financial assistance (Family Equality, 2023). Look into fertility loans if needed. Build contingency plans for what happens if conception takes longer or costs more than expected.

2.4 Insurance Navigation

Insurance coverage for LGBTQ+ family building is inconsistent and often discriminatory. Understanding what's covered and how to advocate matters.

What's usually covered: Prenatal care, birth, and postpartum care are typically covered under maternity benefits if you have insurance.

These are mandated under the Affordable Care Act for most insurance plans. Transgender men sometimes face denials because their gender markers indicate male, triggering automated denials for "gender-inappropriate" services. Fight these denials—they're discriminatory.

What's often not covered: Fertility treatments including IUI and IVF are often excluded from coverage unless you meet "infertility" definitions. Many insurance plans define infertility as 12 months of unsuccessful attempts at pregnancy through intercourse. LGBTQ+ couples obviously don't meet this definition, leading to denials (Perritt, 2017).

Some states mandate fertility coverage: California, Connecticut, Delaware, Hawaii, Illinois, Maryland, Massachusetts, New Hampshire, New Jersey, New York, Rhode Island, and Vermont require some level of fertility treatment coverage. But even in these states, coverage for LGBTQ+ families varies. Some insurers require demonstration of "medical infertility" separate from "social infertility" (not having access to sperm through sex).

Donor sperm costs: Insurance almost never covers donor sperm purchases. You pay out of pocket.

Surrogacy: Insurance for surrogates is complex. The surrogate's health insurance might cover pregnancy, or intended parents might need to purchase separate surrogacy insurance. Read policies carefully—some explicitly exclude surrogacy pregnancies.

Fighting denials: If you receive denials for pregnancy-related care or fertility services you believe should be covered, appeal. Get letters from providers explaining medical necessity. Cite state laws if applicable. Lambda Legal and the National Center for Lesbian Rights provide resources for fighting discriminatory insurance denials (National Center for Lesbian Rights, 2022).

Document everything. Keep copies of policies, denial letters, appeal submissions, and provider letters. Persistence often succeeds because insurance companies count on people giving up.

2.5 Legal Protections

Legal recognition of LGBTQ+ parents varies by state and family configuration. Understanding and securing legal protections prevents catastrophic problems later.

Marriage matters (legally): If you're in a same-sex relationship and married, marriage provides significant legal protections. In most states, a spouse married to someone who gives birth is automatically recognized as a legal parent (though some states still require second-parent adoption). Marriage also affects inheritance, medical decision-making, insurance coverage, and parental rights if relationships end.

If you're not married and could be, consider the legal benefits before conception. If you're opposed to marriage or can't marry (polyamorous relationships, for example), you'll need alternative legal protections.

Second-parent adoption: This legal process allows a non-biological parent to adopt their partner's child without terminating the birth parent's rights. It's often required for non-gestational parents in same-sex couples, though some states now allow both parents to be listed on birth certificates without adoption.

Second-parent adoption provides critical protections: legal parentage if the relationship ends, ability to make medical decisions, inheritance rights, custody if the biological parent dies, and recognition across state lines. Don't skip this even if it seems unnecessary. Laws change and interstate travel happens. Legal parentage matters.

Known donor agreements: If you're using a known sperm donor, get legal agreements in place before conception. These agreements specify that the donor has no parental rights or responsibilities. Without these agreements, known donors can sometimes claim parental rights later, or be held financially responsible for the child (Dempsey, 2013).

Work with attorneys who specialize in LGBTQ+ family law. Donor agreements need careful drafting to hold up legally.

Three or more parents: If you're in a polyamorous family or co-parenting arrangement with more than two adults, legal recognition gets complicated. Very few states recognize more than two legal parents. You'll need creative legal strategies: powers of attorney for medical decisions, guardianship arrangements, wills specifying custody if biological parents die, co-parenting agreements detailing rights and responsibilities.

This legal territory is evolving. Some jurisdictions now recognize three parents in specific circumstances. Work with attorneys familiar with multi-parent families.

Interstate considerations: If you live near state lines or plan to move, understand that parental recognition varies by state. Some states don't fully recognize same-sex parents even post-Obergefell v. Hodges. Carry certified copies of birth certificates, adoption decrees, and court orders establishing parental rights when traveling with your child.

2.6 Fertility Preservation Options

If you're transgender and considering medical transition, or if you're planning to delay parenthood but want to preserve fertility, understanding options matters.

For people with eggs: Egg freezing involves hormone stimulation to produce multiple eggs in one cycle, then surgical retrieval and freezing. It costs $8,000-$15,000 per cycle plus $500-$1,000 annually for storage. Success rates depend on age—eggs frozen in your 20s have much better outcomes than eggs frozen in your late 30s (American Society for Reproductive Medicine, 2023).

Some transgender men freeze eggs before starting testosterone. This provides options for having biological children later using a surrogate or partner. The process requires delaying testosterone for several months and can trigger dysphoria because it involves hyper-feminine hormone states.

For people with sperm: Sperm banking is simpler and cheaper. It costs $1,000-$2,000 initially plus $300-$500 annually for storage. Transgender women can bank sperm before starting estrogen. The process is quick and non-invasive compared to egg freezing.

Ovarian tissue freezing: This experimental option involves surgically removing and freezing ovarian tissue for later reimplantation. It's not widely available and outcomes are uncertain, but it might become more viable as technology advances.

Decision factors: Fertility preservation requires upfront costs for procedures that might never be used. But for transgender people, it's often now or never—testosterone permanently affects fertility in some cases, and estrogen reduces sperm production. Deciding requires balancing immediate transition needs against potential future family desires.

Many transgender people skip fertility preservation because of cost, urgency around transition, or not wanting biological children. That's valid. Others prioritize it despite costs because they know they want the option. Neither choice is wrong.

2.7 Pulling It Together

Consider this composite example: Marcus and Tao started planning their family three years before conception. Marcus is a transgender man. Tao is cisgender male. They knew from the start that Marcus would carry their biological child using Tao's sperm.

They spent the first year saving money—$15,000 for fertility treatments, legal fees, and coverage for Marcus's income loss. They moved from Texas to California to be in a state with better legal protections and non-discrimination laws. They consulted with three attorneys about what legal documents they'd need. They researched trans-friendly fertility clinics.

When Marcus stopped testosterone to prepare for pregnancy, they already had everything lined up: clinic appointments scheduled, known donor agreements in place (they used a friend as a backup option), legal paperwork ready for second-parent adoption. The planning meant that once Marcus was actually pregnant, they could focus on the pregnancy itself rather than scrambling with logistics.

Not everyone can plan this thoroughly. Financial constraints, life circumstances, or urgency around age and fertility sometimes mean proceeding without ideal conditions. But whatever planning you can do now prevents problems later.

2.8 Your Planning Checklist

Family planning for LGBTQ+ people requires thinking through:

- **Family vision**: Who will be parents? Who carries if applicable? What does biological connection mean?
- **Timing**: Age and fertility, financial readiness, career circumstances, relationship stability, legal landscape.
- **Financial planning**: Conception costs, medical costs, legal costs, time off work. Create realistic budgets and backup plans.
- **Insurance**: Understand your coverage. Fight discriminatory denials. Document everything.
- **Legal protections**: Marriage if applicable, second-parent adoption, donor agreements, multi-parent arrangements, interstate considerations.
- **Fertility preservation**: If you're transgender or delaying parenthood, consider egg or sperm banking if financially possible.

Start making lists. Research costs in your area. Talk to attorneys and financial planners. Connect with LGBTQ+ family groups to learn from others' experiences. This planning phase feels tedious but it's the foundation that makes everything else possible.

In Chapter 3.0, we'll talk about choosing your care team—finding providers who understand LGBTQ+ families and can support you through pregnancy and birth. But first, you need clarity on what you're building and how you'll make it happen. That's what this planning phase provides.

Chapter 3.0: Choosing Your Care Team

Finding the right midwife changed everything for Isabella and Carmen. Their first provider seemed fine at the consultation—smiled, said the right things about "being open to all families." But at actual prenatal visits, she consistently directed questions to Isabella (the pregnant partner) while Carmen sat there feeling like furniture. She used "mom" and "dad" language despite their corrections. She seemed confused by their family structure every time they explained it again.

They switched at 20 weeks to a midwife who'd been recommended by other lesbian parents. The difference was immediate. She greeted both of them by name, asked Carmen medical history questions alongside Isabella's, used "mothers" plural naturally, and never once seemed confused about who was who. Carmen attended every prenatal visit feeling like an actual parent instead of a visitor. This matters more than you might think.

Your care team—midwives, obstetricians, nurses, doulas, specialists—will be intimately involved in one of your most vulnerable experiences. Choose people who actually get it, not people who say they get it while treating you like an educational burden.

3.1 What Affirming Care Looks Like

Before we talk about finding affirming providers, let's define what you're looking for. Affirming care means more than tolerance. It means providers who:

Use your language automatically: After you tell them your pronouns, family structure, and preferred terms once, they remember and use them consistently. You shouldn't need to correct pronouns at every visit or re-explain your family composition each time.

Direct care appropriately: If you have a non-gestational partner, affirming providers include them in conversations, ask them questions, direct information to both of you. If you're a transgender man, affirming providers treat you as a man who happens to be pregnant, not as a confused woman.

Know the clinical specifics: Affirming providers understand how testosterone affects pregnancy, what chest-feeding after top surgery involves, how to document gender markers that don't match reproductive capacity, and what legal challenges LGBTQ+ families face. You shouldn't be the one educating them about basic LGBTQ+ reproductive health.

Advocate for you: When hospital staff misgender you or insurance denies coverage unfairly, affirming providers fight on your behalf. They write letters of medical necessity, make phone calls, educate other staff members. They see discrimination as their problem to solve, not yours to tolerate.

Research confirms that LGBTQ+ people who receive affirming care have better health outcomes, higher satisfaction, and increased likelihood of continuing prenatal care (Cahill et al., 2014). This isn't about political correctness—it's about quality care.

3.2 Finding LGBTQ Affirming Providers

Start your search strategically rather than randomly calling practices from your insurance list.

Ask LGBTQ+ communities: Connect with local LGBTQ+ parenting groups, online forums for queer conception, or Pride organizations. Ask who other families recommend. Word of mouth from people with similar identities and experiences is your most reliable guide.

Use specialized directories: Several organizations maintain directories of LGBTQ+-affirming healthcare providers. GLMA (Health Professionals Advancing LGBTQ Equality) has a provider directory searchable by location and specialty. The World Professional Association for Transgender Health lists trans-competent providers. Gay and Lesbian Medical Association maintains referral lists (GLMA, 2023).

Check practice websites and materials: Practices that genuinely prioritize LGBTQ+ care often advertise this on their websites. Look for: inclusive language throughout the site, statements about welcoming all families, photos showing diverse families, mentions of training in LGBTQ+ health, staff pronouns listed.

If a practice website only shows heterosexual couples and uses exclusively "mom and dad" language, that's probably not your best bet. Affirming practices signal their values publicly.

Call and ask directly: When you contact practices, ask specific questions: "Do you have experience with transgender pregnancy?" "How do you document non-gestational parents in your system?" "What's your approach to inclusive language?" "Can you share references from other LGBTQ+ families you've worked with?"

Listen not just to what they say but how they say it. Do they sound comfortable and knowledgeable, or uncertain and defensive? Do they ask clarifying questions to understand your specific needs, or give generic reassurances? Trust your gut about whether they actually understand or are just trying to seem progressive.

3.3 Red Flags and Green Flags

Red flags that signal you should keep looking:

- Provider seems confused or uncomfortable when you explain your family structure
- Repeated pronoun mistakes after corrections

- Directing all questions to the pregnant person while ignoring non-gestational partners
- Comments about "natural" family structures or children "needing" both genders as parents
- Resistance to your language preferences or insistence on using their own terms
- Lack of knowledge about LGBTQ+-specific clinical issues (testosterone and pregnancy, fertility options for queer families, chest-feeding, etc.)
- Requiring extensive education from you about basic LGBTQ+ concepts
- Visible discomfort with your body, identity, or family
- Religious or personal beliefs that conflict with LGBTQ+ families (sometimes stated, sometimes implied)

Green flags that signal good fit:

- Asks what pronouns everyone uses at the start
- Inquires about what terms you prefer for your role, anatomy, and family structure
- Uses inclusive language naturally without it seeming forced
- Includes non-gestational partners in all conversations and decision-making
- Demonstrates knowledge about LGBTQ+ reproductive health specifics
- Provides examples of other LGBTQ+ families they've worked with (without breaking confidentiality)
- Advocates proactively for you with hospital systems, insurance, etc.
- Addresses discrimination when it occurs rather than expecting you to handle it
- Takes your concerns seriously without defensiveness
- Seems genuinely enthusiastic about working with your family

3.4 Questions to Ask Potential Providers

Come to consultations with prepared questions. Don't rely on general impressions—ask specifics.

About experience:

- How many LGBTQ+ families have you worked with?
- Have you cared for transgender men or non-binary people during pregnancy?
- What training have you received in LGBTQ+ perinatal health?
- Can you share references from other LGBTQ+ clients? (They should be able to connect you with past clients who've agreed to talk to potential new clients.)

About clinical approach:

- How do you handle situations where gender markers don't match reproductive anatomy for insurance purposes?
- What's your experience with chest-feeding after top surgery?
- How familiar are you with the effects of testosterone on pregnancy?
- What fertility options do you typically recommend for [your family configuration]?

About documentation and systems:

- How do you document non-gestational partners in your records?
- Can partners attend all appointments and receive all medical information?
- How do you ensure hospital staff use correct names and pronouns during labor and birth?
- What happens if insurance denies coverage due to gender markers?

About birth planning:

- What's your approach to inclusive birth plans?

- How do you prepare hospitals or birth centers for LGBTQ+ families?
- What happens if hospital staff misgender me or my partner during labor?
- Do you have experience with births where the pregnant person doesn't identify as a woman?

About advocacy:

- What do you do if hospital staff or other providers are discriminatory?
- How do you handle situations where my identity conflicts with hospital policies?
- Can you provide letters of medical necessity for insurance appeals?
- What support do you offer for legal parentage issues?

Watch how providers respond. Do they answer confidently with specific examples, or vaguely with platitudes? Do they acknowledge gaps in their knowledge while showing willingness to learn, or get defensive? Do they seem excited about working with your family, or like you're a complicated patient they're reluctantly accepting?

3.5 Care Settings and Considerations

LGBTQ+ families can access affirming care in different settings, each with benefits and challenges.

Hospital birth: Hospitals offer immediate access to medical interventions if needed. But hospitals are large institutions with many staff members, making consistent inclusive care harder. You'll encounter nurses, residents, attending physicians, anesthesiologists, pediatricians—many of whom you've never met. Ensuring everyone uses correct pronouns and understands your family structure requires active effort.

Some hospitals have better LGBTQ+ cultural competency than others. Urban hospitals in progressive areas often have more experience with diverse families. Academic medical centers sometimes have specific training programs. Ask potential providers: How do they prepare hospital staff? What happens when staff make mistakes? Do hospitals have policies protecting LGBTQ+ patients?

Birth centers: Freestanding birth centers often provide more personalized, consistent care with smaller staff teams. You're more likely to build relationships with everyone who'll attend your birth. Birth centers typically embrace midwifery model care that prioritizes patient-centered approaches—this often translates to better LGBTQ+ care.

But birth centers serve lower-risk pregnancies. If complications arise, you'll transfer to a hospital where you haven't established relationships. And not all birth centers are LGBTQ+-affirming—some have religious affiliations that create complications.

Home birth: Home birth offers maximum control over your environment and who's present. You choose your midwife carefully, and that person (plus maybe one assistant) is your entire care team. Many LGBTQ+ families love home birth because they avoid institutional discrimination entirely.

But home birth requires careful risk assessment. It's safest for low-risk pregnancies with easy access to hospital backup if needed. And not all home birth midwives are LGBTQ+-affirming—some have conservative beliefs that conflict with queer families.

Choosing your setting: Consider your risk level, comfort with medical settings, importance of control versus immediate intervention access, and where you'll find the most affirming care. All three settings can work for LGBTQ+ families if you find the right providers.

3.6 Doula Support

Doulas provide continuous physical, emotional, and informational support during pregnancy, labor, and postpartum. For LGBTQ+

families, doulas can be especially helpful as advocates and buffers against discrimination.

What doulas do: They attend prenatal appointments, provide education, suggest comfort measures during labor, advocate for your preferences with medical staff, support partners in supporting you, and continue care postpartum. Doulas don't replace midwives or obstetricians—they complement medical care with non-medical support.

Research shows that doula support reduces cesarean rates, improves birth satisfaction, and increases successful feeding initiation (Bohren et al., 2017). For LGBTQ+ families specifically, doulas who understand your identity and family structure can help ensure respectful care throughout.

Finding LGBTQ+ affirming doulas: Look for doulas who specifically advertise LGBTQ+ competency. Some doulas specialize in transgender pregnancy support, others in helping non-gestational partners feel actively involved, others in navigating discrimination in healthcare settings.

Interview doulas carefully. Ask about their experience with families like yours, their approach to advocacy, how they handle discrimination, what language they use, and whether they've received specific training in LGBTQ+ issues. Many doulas offer free or reduced-cost consultations.

Doula benefits for specific situations:

- Transgender men often appreciate doulas who can advocate around pronouns and names with hospital staff
- Lesbian couples benefit from doulas who actively involve non-gestational partners rather than assuming only the pregnant person needs support
- Single parents by choice need doulas who provide partner-level support without romantic assumptions

- Polyamorous families benefit from doulas who understand multiple support people and complex family structures

3.7 Building Your Wider Support Network

Beyond your medical care team, you need emotional and practical support throughout pregnancy, birth, and early parenting.

LGBTQ+ parenting groups: Connect with others navigating similar experiences. Online communities like queer conception groups, transgender pregnancy forums, and lesbian parents' networks provide space to ask questions, share resources, and feel less alone. Local in-person groups offer practical support and potential lasting friendships.

Mental health support: Consider working with a therapist who understands LGBTQ+ identities and reproductive experiences. Pregnancy triggers unexpected emotions. Navigating discrimination is stressful. Partners sometimes struggle with their roles and feelings. Having mental health support prevents problems from becoming crises.

Legal support: Consult with attorneys specializing in LGBTQ+ family law early in pregnancy. Don't wait until problems arise. Get legal documents in place for parental recognition, prepare for potential insurance battles, understand your rights if discrimination occurs.

Practical help: Identify who will provide practical support—meals, childcare for older children, help with household tasks. LGBTQ+ families sometimes lack automatic support from biological families due to rejection or complicated relationships. Building intentional support networks matters more.

Chosen family: Many LGBTQ+ people have created families of choice—close friends who function as family. Include these people in your pregnancy and birth planning if they're willing and capable. Chosen family can fill gaps that biological family might not.

3.8 When to Change Providers

Sometimes you choose wrong initially, or providers who seemed fine early on show problematic behaviors later. Don't stay with inadequate care out of inertia or guilt.

Reasons to consider switching:

- Repeated pronoun or name mistakes despite corrections
- Consistent exclusion of non-gestational partners
- Comments that feel dismissive of your identity or family
- Lack of knowledge about LGBTQ+-specific issues with no effort to learn
- Passive response to discrimination from other staff
- Your gut feeling that something is off
- Increased stress around appointments rather than comfort
- Provider making your pregnancy about their learning rather than your care

How to switch: You can change providers at any point during pregnancy. Some practices have policies about accepting new patients after certain gestational ages, but many will accommodate transfers. Be direct about why you're leaving if you're comfortable—your feedback might improve care for future LGBTQ+ families. If you're not comfortable explaining, you don't owe anyone justification.

Get copies of your medical records to bring to your new provider. This ensures continuity of care and avoids repeating tests unnecessarily.

Finding better care: Use the same strategies from section 3.2 but with added experience. You now know what doesn't work. Ask more pointed questions. Trust your instincts faster. Most LGBTQ+ families who switch providers report relief at finding better care, wishing only that they'd switched sooner.

3.9 Moving Forward

Consider this composite scenario: Riley, a non-binary person, interviewed five different practices before choosing their midwife. The first three felt awkward—providers stumbling over pronouns, asking invasive questions about their genitals in the consultation (before any medical need), seeming uncertain how to document their gender in records. The fourth practice seemed better but didn't have experience with non-binary pregnancy and was honest that Riley would be teaching them.

The fifth practice had a midwife who lit up when Riley explained their identity and pregnancy plans. She'd worked with two other non-binary pregnant people and several transgender men. She immediately asked Riley's pronouns and what terms they wanted used. She explained how they document gender neutrally in their system and showed Riley examples of birth plans for non-binary clients. She asked smart questions about Riley's specific needs rather than making assumptions.

Riley left that consultation knowing they'd found the right fit. And throughout pregnancy, that midwife proved it—advocating with insurance when claims were denied, preparing the hospital for Riley's specific needs, handling Riley's dysphoria compassionately, and treating Riley's pregnancy as exactly what it was: a non-binary person growing a baby.

That's what you're looking for. Keep searching until you find it.

3.10 Essential Points to Remember

Choosing your care team sets the tone for your entire pregnancy experience. Prioritize finding affirming providers over staying with convenient but inadequate care. Use LGBTQ+ community recommendations, ask direct questions, watch for red and green flags, and don't hesitate to switch if needed.

Your care team should include medical providers (midwives or obstetricians), potentially a doula, mental health support, legal support, and practical help from community and chosen family.

Build this network intentionally rather than assuming it will materialize when needed.

In Chapter 4.0, we'll cover understanding your body and fertility—the biological foundations you need before moving into specific conception strategies in Chapters 5.0-9.0. But first, make sure you have the right people supporting you through this journey.

Chapter 4.0: Understanding Your Body and Fertility

Here's something nobody tells you until you're actively trying to get pregnant: understanding fertility is way more complicated than high school health class suggested. And for LGBTQ+ people, it gets even more layered because the standard fertility information assumes you're having penis-in-vagina sex every month, which obviously doesn't apply to most of our situations.

You need to understand how your specific body works, how hormones affect fertility across different identities, what timing actually matters, and when to worry versus when to be patient. This chapter covers the biological foundations that inform everything in the conception chapters that follow.

4.1 Reproductive Anatomy Basics

Let's start with the fundamental biology, because you need this foundation before we get into the complications.

For bodies with ovaries and uteruses: Fertility depends on having viable eggs, functional ovaries that release them, open fallopian tubes for fertilization to occur, and a uterus that can support implantation and pregnancy. Every month (roughly), one ovary releases an egg in a process called ovulation. That egg lives for about 12-24 hours. If sperm are present in the fallopian tube during that window, fertilization might happen. The fertilized egg then travels to the uterus and implants in the uterine lining.

This process requires specific hormone patterns. The hypothalamus and pituitary gland in your brain signal your ovaries to mature eggs and produce estrogen. Rising estrogen triggers ovulation. After ovulation, the empty follicle becomes the corpus luteum, which produces progesterone to prepare the uterine lining for potential pregnancy. If no pregnancy occurs, hormone levels drop and menstruation happens.

For bodies with testes and sperm production: Fertility depends on producing viable sperm and having functioning delivery systems. Sperm production happens continuously in the testes, taking about 74 days from start to finish. Mature sperm are stored in the epididymis until ejaculation. During ejaculation, sperm mix with fluid from the seminal vesicles and prostate to create semen.

Sperm production requires specific hormone signals from the brain and particular temperature conditions (which is why testes hang outside the body—they need to be slightly cooler than core body temperature). Once ejaculated into a vagina, sperm can survive for 3-5 days in fertile cervical mucus, waiting for an egg to be released.

Why this matters for LGBTQ+ families: Understanding these basics helps you make informed decisions about conception methods. If you're using fresh sperm from a known donor, timing matters because sperm survive several days. If you're using frozen sperm, timing matters even more because frozen sperm have shorter survival. If you're a transgender man with a uterus, you need to know that testosterone suppresses ovulation but doesn't eliminate it entirely.

4.2 How Hormones Affect Fertility

Hormones control everything about fertility. Understanding them helps you optimize timing and recognize when something might be off.

The menstrual cycle: A typical cycle lasts 24-35 days, though there's wide variation. The first day of bleeding is cycle day one. During the follicular phase (roughly days 1-14), estrogen rises as follicles develop. Ovulation typically happens around day 14 in a 28-day cycle, triggered by a surge in luteinizing hormone (LH). The luteal phase (days 15-28) involves progesterone production. If pregnancy doesn't occur, both estrogen and progesterone drop, triggering menstruation.

Fertility is highest in the few days before ovulation and the day of ovulation itself. This is called the fertile window—roughly five to six days each cycle when conception is possible (Wilcox et al., 1995).

Testosterone's effects: Testosterone therapy suppresses ovulation in most transgender men, but not universally or permanently (Light et al., 2014). Some transgender men continue to ovulate occasionally even on testosterone. Stopping testosterone usually restores ovulation within a few months, but there's individual variation. Some people resume cycling immediately. Others take six months or more.

Testosterone doesn't permanently damage fertility in most cases, but long-term effects aren't fully studied. If you're a transgender man planning pregnancy, expect that stopping testosterone will eventually restore fertility, but the timeline varies.

Age-related changes: Fertility declines with age, particularly for people with ovaries. This decline accelerates after age 35 and becomes steep after 40. By age 40, fertility is about half of what it was at age 30 (American Society for Reproductive Medicine, 2012). This happens because egg quantity and quality both decrease over time.

For people with sperm, age affects fertility less dramatically but still matters. Sperm quality declines gradually after age 40, and older paternal age is associated with slightly increased risks of certain conditions in offspring.

Other hormone considerations: Conditions like polycystic ovary syndrome (PCOS), thyroid disorders, and hormonal imbalances affect fertility. PCOS causes irregular ovulation or anovulation (no ovulation), making conception timing difficult. Thyroid problems can prevent ovulation or cause early miscarriage. If your cycles are very irregular or absent, hormone evaluation makes sense before actively trying to conceive.

4.3 Fertility Awareness and Tracking

Knowing when ovulation happens maximizes your chances of conception and minimizes costs if you're buying sperm or paying for procedures.

Tracking methods: Several approaches help identify your fertile window:

Basal body temperature (BBT): Your resting body temperature rises slightly (0.5-1°F) after ovulation due to progesterone. By tracking temperature daily before getting out of bed, you can confirm that ovulation occurred. But BBT tells you after the fact—it's better for confirming ovulation patterns than predicting fertile days in real time.

Cervical mucus monitoring: As ovulation approaches, cervical mucus changes from thick and sticky to clear, slippery, and stretchy (like raw egg whites). This fertile-quality mucus helps sperm survive and travel. Learning to observe and interpret cervical mucus gives you advance warning that ovulation is approaching.

Ovulation predictor kits (OPKs): These detect the LH surge that triggers ovulation, giving you 12-36 hours notice before an egg is released. OPKs are useful for timing insemination attempts. You test daily during the days you expect ovulation (typically days 10-16 of your cycle), looking for the surge.

Fertility awareness apps: Apps like Kindara, Fertility Friend, or Clue help track cycles, symptoms, and test results. They can predict fertile windows based on your data, though predictions are only as accurate as your tracking consistency.

Calendar method: If your cycles are regular, you can estimate ovulation as 14 days before your expected period. This is less reliable than other methods because cycle length varies, but it's a starting point.

For LGBTQ+ families using donor sperm or clinical procedures, accurate tracking saves money. Every insemination attempt costs hundreds to thousands of dollars. Pinpointing ovulation means you're not wasting resources on poorly-timed attempts.

4.4 Testosterone and Pregnancy Planning

If you're a transgender man or non-binary person who's been on testosterone and wants to become pregnant, you need specific information about stopping hormones and what to expect.

Stopping testosterone: Most healthcare providers recommend stopping testosterone at least three months before actively trying to conceive, allowing time for your cycle to return and for any residual testosterone to clear your system (Obedin-Maliver & Makadon, 2016). Some people conceive successfully sooner. Others take longer to resume cycling.

The process of stopping testosterone triggers resumption of menstruation for most people, though timing varies. Expect irregular cycles initially as your body readjusts. Some people experience cramping, mood changes, and other menstrual symptoms they might not have had for years.

Managing dysphoria: Stopping testosterone often increases dysphoria. Menstruation returns. Secondary sex characteristics that testosterone suppressed (like breast tissue) become more prominent. Your voice won't change back, and facial hair won't disappear, but other changes can feel distressing.

Plan ahead for dysphoria management: connect with a therapist, build support systems, remind yourself this is temporary and purposeful. Some transgender men find it helps to view pregnancy as an intensely male experience they're uniquely capable of—growing their child in their own body. Others frame it as a medical process they're undergoing to achieve a goal. Find the mental framework that works for you.

Pregnancy while on testosterone: Accidentally becoming pregnant while on testosterone is possible if you're having sex that could result in pregnancy. Testosterone is not reliable birth control. If this happens, stop testosterone immediately and seek prenatal care. Limited research exists on testosterone exposure in early pregnancy, but available evidence suggests that stopping testosterone as soon as pregnancy is discovered doesn't typically cause problems (Light et al., 2014).

Post-pregnancy considerations: After birth, you can resume testosterone once you're done chest-feeding (if applicable) or immediately if you're not planning to feed. Some transgender men restart testosterone very quickly postpartum to minimize dysphoria. Others wait months if they're chest-feeding. There's no single right timeline.

4.5 Fertility Evaluation Timing

When should you seek fertility evaluation versus continuing to try on your own? The standard medical advice doesn't quite fit LGBTQ+ families.

Traditional guidelines: Heterosexual couples are typically advised to try for 12 months (if under 35) or six months (if over 35) before seeking fertility evaluation. This assumes regular, unprotected intercourse throughout.

Modified guidelines for LGBTQ+ families: If you're using donor sperm and timed insemination attempts, consider seeking evaluation after:

- Six cycles of well-timed attempts if you're under 35
- Three to four cycles if you're over 35

- Sooner if you have known fertility concerns (irregular cycles, PCOS, previous fertility problems, history of pelvic infections, endometriosis)

Why earlier than heterosexual couples? Because each attempt costs money and emotional energy. If something is preventing conception, you want to know sooner rather than later (Ethics Committee of the American Society for Reproductive Medicine, 2013).

What evaluation involves: Basic fertility workup includes:

- Hormone testing (FSH, LH, estradiol, AMH, thyroid hormones)
- Ovarian reserve testing to assess egg quantity
- Ultrasound to check uterus and ovaries
- Sometimes HSG (hysterosalpingogram) to check if fallopian tubes are open
- Semen analysis if using a known donor

For transgender men, evaluation might include assessing how fully your cycle has returned after stopping testosterone and whether ovulation is occurring.

For gay male couples: Fertility evaluation focuses on sperm quality if you're providing sperm for IVF. Standard semen analysis checks sperm count, motility (movement), and morphology (shape).

4.6 When Bodies Don't Cooperate

Fertility challenges affect LGBTQ+ families just like anyone else. Understanding common issues helps you recognize when to seek help.

Ovulation disorders: PCOS is the most common cause of ovulation problems, affecting about 10% of women of reproductive age (Azziz et al., 2016). It causes irregular or absent ovulation, making conception timing difficult. Treatment often involves medications like letrozole or clomiphene to induce ovulation.

Blocked fallopian tubes: Infections, endometriosis, or previous surgeries can block fallopian tubes, preventing sperm and egg from meeting. This requires either surgical repair or moving to IVF (which bypasses tubes entirely).

Uterine issues: Fibroids, polyps, or structural abnormalities in the uterus can prevent implantation. Surgical treatment might be necessary.

Sperm problems: Low sperm count, poor motility, or abnormal morphology affect conception chances. If you're using a known donor whose sperm has problems, you might need IUI or IVF rather than home insemination.

Unexplained infertility: Sometimes all testing comes back normal but pregnancy still doesn't happen. This is frustrating but relatively common. Treatment often involves trying IUI or IVF even without a clear diagnosis.

Consider this composite example: Maria and Elena tried at-home insemination for eight cycles with consistently well-timed attempts. Nothing. They sought fertility evaluation and discovered that Maria had blocked fallopian tubes from a previous undiagnosed chlamydia infection. IUI wouldn't work for her—she needed IVF. Learning this after eight months of expensive, failed attempts was frustrating, but it redirected them toward an approach that could actually succeed.

The lesson: if conception isn't happening after several well-timed attempts, get evaluated. Don't assume your body will eventually cooperate.

4.7 Mental Health and Conception Readiness

Fertility isn't just physical. Your mental health affects conception readiness and your ability to handle the process.

Stress and fertility: Research on stress and fertility is mixed, but chronic high stress can affect ovulation and overall health (Louis et al., 2011). More importantly, the conception process itself creates stress—especially when it takes longer than expected or involves medical intervention.

Build stress management strategies before you start trying: therapy, meditation, exercise, support groups, whatever works for you. The process will test your emotional resilience.

Relationship readiness: If you're partnered, how solid is your relationship? Conception challenges strain relationships. Pregnancy and parenting are intense. Starting from a strong foundation matters.

If there are unresolved conflicts, consider couples counseling before conception. If the relationship is new, consider whether you're rushing into parenthood before you've built adequate stability.

Individual mental health: Untreated depression, anxiety, trauma, or other mental health conditions affect your capacity to handle the demands of conception, pregnancy, and parenting. This doesn't mean you can't become a parent—it means you need treatment and support systems in place.

Work with mental health providers who understand LGBTQ+ identities. Some therapists specialize in reproductive mental health and can help you navigate conception challenges, pregnancy, and postpartum periods.

Dysphoria considerations: For transgender and non-binary people, pregnancy involves intense physical changes that can trigger dysphoria. Assess realistically: Can you handle menstruation returning if you've been on testosterone? Can you handle your body becoming more curvy and "feminine" during pregnancy? Can you handle being misgendered constantly as pregnancy becomes visible?

These aren't reasons not to pursue pregnancy—plenty of transgender men and non-binary people navigate this successfully. But they're factors to plan for with therapist support and coping strategies in place.

4.8 Pulling Knowledge Together

Understanding your body and fertility creates the foundation for making informed conception decisions. You need to know:

- How your reproductive anatomy functions
- How hormones control fertility and when your fertile window occurs
- How to track ovulation accurately
- How testosterone affects fertility and what stopping it involves
- When to seek fertility evaluation versus continuing independent attempts
- What common fertility challenges look like
- Whether you're mentally and emotionally ready for this process

This knowledge shapes everything in Chapters 5.0 through 9.0, where we cover specific conception methods for different family configurations. Lesbian couples timing insemination need to understand fertile windows. Transgender men need to understand how stopping testosterone affects their bodies. Gay male couples using surrogacy need to understand sperm quality factors. Everyone needs to understand when persistence makes sense versus when medical help is necessary.

Think about your own body. What do you know about your fertility? What gaps exist in your knowledge? What tracking methods would work for your lifestyle? What mental health support do you need in place?

4.9 Moving Into Conception Planning

With understanding of bodies and fertility established, you're ready for specific conception guidance. Chapter 5.0 covers options for lesbian and queer couples. Chapter 6.0 addresses transgender men and non-binary people. Chapter 7.0 explains surrogacy for gay male couples. Chapter 8.0 discusses alternative family configurations.

Chapter 9.0 covers what happens when conception takes longer than expected.

Each conception path involves different considerations, but all build on the biological foundations covered here. Your body is the starting point. Understanding how it works—and doesn't work—empowers you to make strategic decisions about conception methods, timing, and when to seek help.

Part Two: Conception Pathways

Chapter 5.0: Conception for Lesbian Couples

Isabella wanted to carry. Jasmine wanted to carry. They both wanted biological connection to their future children. They'd been together five years, married for two, and ready to start their family. But the question of who would go first consumed months of conversations, spreadsheets analyzing pros and cons, and eventually some arguments that felt bigger than they should have.

This is where straight couples have it easier—biology makes the decision for them. Lesbian couples get to choose, which sounds empowering until you're actually doing it and realizing that every choice means someone waits.

This chapter covers the full spectrum of conception options for lesbian and queer female couples: deciding who carries, choosing between known and anonymous donors, at-home insemination methods, clinical IUI, IVF options including reciprocal IVF, working with fertility clinics, and legal considerations. If you're a lesbian couple or queer women planning pregnancy, this is your roadmap.

5.1 Deciding Who Carries

If both partners have uteruses and both want to carry, you need a decision framework that works for your specific situation.

Age and fertility considerations: If one partner is significantly older or approaching 35, that person might go first since fertility declines with age. Waiting could mean needing fertility treatments later. Some couples alternate—the older partner carries first, then the younger partner carries subsequent children.

Health factors: Pre-existing health conditions, medications incompatible with pregnancy, or known fertility issues might influence who carries. If one partner has PCOS or irregular cycles, the other might have an easier time conceiving.

Career timing: Whose career better accommodates pregnancy and parental leave right now? This isn't about one career being more important—it's practical assessment of timing, leave policies, and flexibility. Some couples prioritize the partner whose job offers better parental leave or more stability.

Desire intensity: Sometimes one partner wants the pregnancy experience more intensely. This might be enough reason on its own. Resentment builds if the less interested partner carries while the more interested partner watches.

Biological connection options: Reciprocal IVF (covered in section 5.6) allows both partners biological connection when one carries using the other's eggs. This option requires IVF costs but provides a solution if biological connection matters deeply to both partners.

Just making a choice: Sometimes analysis paralysis sets in. You've considered every factor and still can't decide. At some point, someone has to go first. Some couples flip a coin. Others set a deadline for deciding and stick to it. Neither approach is wrong if you've both genuinely considered the options.

Think about what feels fair in your relationship. Fair doesn't always mean equal. Fair means you both feel respected and considered.

5.2 Known Versus Anonymous Donors

Sperm has to come from somewhere. You'll either know the donor personally or use anonymous donor sperm from a sperm bank. Both options have benefits and complications.

Known donor benefits:

- Free or much cheaper than purchasing sperm
- Known medical history, personality, appearance
- Potential ongoing relationship between donor and child
- Child knows biological origins
- Some families value this extended connection

Known donor complications:

- Legal risks if donor agreements aren't properly executed
- Potential for donor to claim parental rights or be held financially responsible
- Relationship complications if donor becomes too involved or not involved enough
- Risk of relationship breakdown affecting child
- Requires STI testing and often fertility evaluation
- Logistics of coordinating conception timing with donor's schedule

Anonymous donor benefits:

- Clear legal boundaries—donor has no parental rights or responsibilities
- No relationship complications to navigate
- Professional screening for genetic conditions, infectious diseases, fertility
- Extensive donor profiles with medical history, photos, personal essays
- Can purchase multiple vials from same donor for genetic siblings
- Available on your timeline without coordinating with another person's schedule

Anonymous donor complications:

- Expensive ($500-$1,000 per vial plus shipping)
- Limited information about donor compared to someone you know

- Child won't know biological father unless donor is "open" (identity-release donor who can be contacted when child turns 18)
- Sperm banks can run out of particular donors, making genetic siblings complicated
- Requires selecting donor based on profiles rather than personal knowledge

Legal considerations: If you use a known donor, get legal agreements drafted by an attorney specializing in reproductive law. These agreements must clearly state that the donor has no parental rights or responsibilities. Without proper legal documents, known donors can potentially claim paternity rights or be held financially responsible for child support (Dempsey, 2013).

Anonymous donor sperm from reputable sperm banks comes with legal clarity—donors sign away all parental rights, and sperm banks handle the legal framework.

5.3 At Home Insemination Methods

Many lesbian couples start with at-home insemination because it's cheaper and more private than clinical procedures. Success rates for at-home insemination with good timing are similar to IUI in fertile women (Ferrara et al., 2018).

The basic process:

1. Track ovulation using methods from Chapter 4.0
2. Obtain fresh sperm from known donor or thawed frozen sperm from sperm bank
3. Insert sperm as close to cervix as possible
4. Rest for 20-30 minutes to allow sperm to travel through cervix
5. Wait approximately two weeks and test for pregnancy

Methods for insertion:

Needleless syringe: Most common approach. Use a sterile needleless syringe (typically 5-10ml) to draw up semen, insert the syringe tip into the vagina near the cervix, and slowly push the plunger to deposit semen. You can purchase syringes designed specifically for this purpose or use standard needleless syringes from pharmacies.

Cervical cap method: Some people use a cervical cap or menstrual disc to hold semen against the cervix. Place semen in the cap, insert it over the cervix, and leave it in place for several hours. This keeps semen in contact with the cervix longer.

Timing considerations: Inseminate during your fertile window—the five days before ovulation through the day of ovulation. If using fresh sperm from a known donor, inseminate the day before expected ovulation and/or the day of ovulation. If using frozen sperm, inseminate as close to ovulation as possible since frozen sperm have shorter survival times (12-24 hours versus 3-5 days for fresh).

Success rates: With good timing and no fertility issues, at-home insemination has success rates of about 10-15% per cycle, similar to natural conception rates for heterosexual couples (Ferrara et al., 2018). Success rates are higher with fresh sperm versus frozen, and with more than one insemination per cycle.

Safety considerations:

- Use sterile equipment
- If using known donor, ensure recent STI testing
- Wash hands thoroughly
- Don't introduce anything non-sterile into vagina
- Follow proper handling for frozen sperm (thaw according to sperm bank instructions)

When at-home insemination makes sense: If you're young (under 35), have regular cycles, no known fertility issues, and want to avoid medical intervention, at-home insemination is a reasonable starting point. Most couples try 3-6 cycles at home before moving to clinical options.

5.4 Clinical IUI

Intrauterine insemination (IUI) is a clinical procedure where washed sperm is inserted directly into the uterus using a thin catheter. IUI bypasses the cervix, placing sperm closer to the fallopian tubes where fertilization occurs.

The IUI process:

1. Cycle monitoring through fertility clinic—blood work and ultrasounds to track follicle development
2. Ovulation trigger shot (HCG) when follicles are mature, causing ovulation within 36 hours
3. IUI procedure performed 24-36 hours after trigger shot
4. Sperm is "washed" to separate the highest-quality sperm from seminal fluid
5. Sperm is inserted through catheter into uterus
6. Wait approximately two weeks and test for pregnancy

IUI versus at-home insemination: IUI offers several advantages:

- Sperm is placed directly in uterus, bypassing cervical mucus that might hinder sperm movement
- Sperm washing selects the most motile sperm
- Precise timing through monitoring and trigger shots
- Medical supervision throughout

Success rates for IUI are slightly higher than at-home insemination—about 15-20% per cycle in women under 35 without fertility issues (Matorras et al., 2015). Success rates decrease with age and fertility problems.

Costs: IUI costs $300-$1,000 per cycle depending on location and clinic, plus monitoring costs (ultrasounds and bloodwork) which might add another $200-$500 per cycle. Add sperm costs ($500-$1,000 per vial).

When IUI makes sense: Move to IUI if:

- At-home insemination hasn't worked after several cycles
- You have mild fertility issues (slightly irregular ovulation, cervical mucus problems)
- You're over 35 and want to maximize efficiency
- You want medical monitoring and support throughout the process
- You have insurance coverage that pays for IUI but not at-home attempts

5.5 IVF for Lesbian Couples

In vitro fertilization (IVF) involves retrieving eggs from ovaries, fertilizing them with sperm in a lab, growing embryos for several days, and transferring one or more embryos back into the uterus.

The IVF process:

1. Ovarian stimulation with injectable hormones for 8-14 days to produce multiple eggs
2. Monitoring through frequent ultrasounds and bloodwork
3. Trigger shot when eggs are mature
4. Egg retrieval procedure (under sedation) 36 hours after trigger
5. Sperm fertilizes eggs in the lab
6. Embryos develop for 3-5 days
7. Embryo transfer into uterus
8. Wait approximately two weeks and test for pregnancy

When IVF is recommended:

- Failed IUI cycles (typically 3-6 attempts)
- Blocked or damaged fallopian tubes

- Severe fertility issues (poor ovarian reserve, ovulation disorders not responding to medications)
- Age-related fertility decline
- Desire to do preimplantation genetic testing on embryos
- Reciprocal IVF (see section 5.6)

Success rates: IVF success rates depend heavily on age. For women under 35, success rates are approximately 50% per embryo transfer. Rates decline to about 35% for women 35-37, and continue declining with age (Society for Assisted Reproductive Technology, 2022).

Costs: IVF costs $12,000-$25,000 per cycle including medications, monitoring, egg retrieval, lab fees, and embryo transfer. Add sperm costs. Most people need multiple cycles to achieve pregnancy, though many freeze extra embryos from one retrieval for future use.

Advantages over IUI: IVF allows genetic testing of embryos before transfer, increases success rates per attempt, and creates frozen embryos for future children. For couples with specific fertility challenges or poor IUI outcomes, IVF offers better chances.

5.6 Reciprocal IVF

Reciprocal IVF is a variation where one partner provides eggs and the other partner carries the pregnancy. Both partners have biological and gestational connections to the child—one genetic, one through pregnancy.

How reciprocal IVF works:

1. One partner undergoes ovarian stimulation and egg retrieval (the genetic parent)
2. Her eggs are fertilized with donor sperm
3. Resulting embryos are transferred to the other partner's uterus (the gestational parent)
4. The gestational partner carries the pregnancy

This creates unique connection: the genetic parent contributed her DNA, and the gestational parent grew the baby in her body. Both partners are mothers in distinct biological ways.

Why choose reciprocal IVF:

- Both partners want biological connection to children
- Genetic parent has fertility challenges making conception difficult but produces good quality eggs
- Gestational parent has excellent uterine environment for carrying pregnancy
- Emotional importance of both partners being biologically involved
- Creates a shared biological bond that feels significant to the couple

Costs and considerations: Reciprocal IVF costs the same as standard IVF ($12,000-$25,000) since the process is identical except the embryo goes into a different uterus. Both partners need medical screening—genetic parent for ovarian reserve and response to medications, gestational partner for uterine health and hormone responsiveness.

Both partners are medically involved: genetic parent goes through stimulation and retrieval, gestational parent takes estrogen and progesterone to prepare uterus for transfer and support early pregnancy.

Legal considerations: In most states, the gestational parent is legally recognized as the birth parent. The genetic parent must typically complete second-parent adoption to establish legal parentage, even though she provided the egg. Work with attorneys familiar with reciprocal IVF to ensure both parents have legal recognition.

Consider Elena and Jasmine's decision (a composite example): After months of discussing who would carry, they discovered reciprocal IVF. Elena would provide eggs—she had excellent ovarian reserve testing but a history of endometriosis that complicated implantation. Jasmine would carry—her uterus was perfect but she had lower ovarian reserve. Reciprocal IVF let them both participate biologically. The first transfer worked. When their daughter was born, Elena felt connected through genetics and Jasmine through pregnancy. Both felt like mothers from the start.

5.7 Working With Fertility Clinics

Fertility clinics provide IUI and IVF services. Choosing the right clinic matters for both success rates and experience as a lesbian couple.

Finding LGBTQ-affirming clinics: Not all fertility clinics are equally welcoming to lesbian couples. Some are actively affirming. Others are technically willing to treat you but make assumptions or use language that feels exclusionary. Look for clinics that:

- Explicitly advertise LGBTQ+ family building services on their website
- Have intake forms and systems designed for same-sex couples
- Include both partners in all conversations and decision-making
- Use inclusive language naturally
- Have prior experience with lesbian couples (ask for approximate numbers)

Ask other lesbian parents for recommendations. Check online reviews from LGBTQ+ families. Interview multiple clinics before choosing.

Questions to ask potential clinics:

- How many lesbian couples do you work with annually?
- How do you ensure both partners are included in care?
- What's your success rate for women in my age group?
- Do you offer reciprocal IVF?

- How do you handle insurance for same-sex couples?
- What's your approach if initial treatments don't work?
- Can you provide references from other lesbian couples?

Insurance navigation: Many insurance plans don't cover IUI or IVF for lesbian couples because you don't meet "infertility" definitions requiring 12 months of failed intercourse. Some states mandate coverage that includes same-sex couples. Some clinics help with insurance appeals. Get clarity upfront about costs and coverage.

Partner involvement: Ensure the clinic treats both partners as parents from the start. The non-gestational partner should receive medical updates, attend appointments, participate in decisions, and be included in all communication. If a clinic defaults to only talking to the person undergoing treatment, that's a red flag.

5.8 Donor Selection Strategies

If you're using anonymous donor sperm, you'll spend significant time reviewing donor profiles. This process feels both weighty (you're choosing half of your child's genetics) and absurd (you're picking someone from a catalog based on baby photos and essay answers).

What sperm banks provide: Donor profiles typically include:

- Medical history for donor and extended family
- Physical characteristics (height, weight, eye color, hair color and texture, ethnicity, blood type)
- Education and occupation
- Childhood and adult photos
- Audio or video recordings
- Written essays about personality, interests, values
- Staff impressions of donor
- Genetic testing results
- Information about donor's availability

Identity-release versus anonymous: Some donors are "open" or "identity-release," meaning your child can contact them when they turn 18. Anonymous donors cannot be contacted. Think about whether your child knowing their biological origins matters to you.

Selection factors: Couples prioritize different things:

- Physical resemblance to non-genetic parent
- Ethnicity and cultural background
- Intelligence and education level
- Personality traits
- Medical history
- Artistic or athletic abilities
- Open versus anonymous status

Some couples seek donors who match the non-genetic parent's appearance so the child looks like both mothers. Others prioritize ethnic heritage if they want their child to share that identity. Others care most about health history and intelligence.

Practical considerations: Popular donors sell out quickly. If you want genetic siblings, purchase multiple vials from the same donor upfront and keep them in storage. Sperm banks charge storage fees ($300-$500 annually) but this ensures availability.

Consider buying more vials than you think you'll need. Conception might take multiple cycles. You might want multiple children. Donors retire from programs or sell out.

5.9 Legal Protections

Even with conception methods established, legal protections matter. Get these in place before conception.

Second-parent adoption: In most states, the non-genetic parent must complete second-parent adoption to establish legal parentage. This applies even if you're married. Start researching the process in your state before conception so you know timing and requirements.

Donor agreements: If using a known donor, legal agreements are essential (covered in section 5.2). Work with attorneys who specialize in reproductive law to draft agreements that protect your family.

Both names on birth certificate: Some states allow both mothers' names on the original birth certificate. Others require second-parent adoption first. Understand your state's requirements.

Interstate considerations: Parental recognition varies by state. If you live near state lines, travel frequently, or might move, understand that some states don't fully recognize same-sex parents despite federal marriage equality.

5.10 Your Conception Plan

With all these options, create a specific plan:

1. **Decision on who carries**: Make this choice with input from both partners considering age, health, career, desire, and fairness.
2. **Donor selection**: Known versus anonymous, and if anonymous, specific donor selection based on your values and priorities.
3. **Method choice**: Start with at-home insemination, or go straight to IUI or IVF? This depends on age, finances, fertility status, and efficiency preferences.
4. **Timeline and budget**: How many cycles will you try with each method? What's your financial budget? How long are you willing to continue before trying different approaches?
5. **Legal protections**: Research second-parent adoption requirements and timeline. If using known donor, get agreements drafted before conception.

In Chapter 6.0, we'll cover conception for transgender men and non-binary people. Chapter 7.0 addresses surrogacy for gay male couples. Chapter 8.0 covers alternative family configurations. And

Chapter 9.0 discusses what to do when conception takes longer than expected.

For now, understand your options as a lesbian couple, make strategic decisions based on your specific circumstances, and build your path forward intentionally.

5.11 Key Takeaways

Lesbian couples have multiple conception options, from at-home insemination through reciprocal IVF. Decisions involve who carries, donor selection, method choice, and legal protections. Success requires understanding your options, choosing affirming providers, planning strategically, and securing legal parental recognition for both parents.

Most lesbian couples conceive successfully within 6-12 cycles of well-timed attempts if starting before age 35 without fertility issues. Older age or fertility challenges might require moving to IVF sooner. Throughout the process, ensure both partners stay actively involved and emotionally supported.

Chapter 6.0: Conception for Transgender Men

Marcus stopped his testosterone on a Tuesday. He'd been on testosterone for six years—six years of his voice dropping, facial hair growing, fat redistributing, muscles developing. Six years of finally feeling at home in his body. And now he was stopping. To get pregnant.

The dysphoria hit within weeks. His period returned after three months. He cried in the bathroom, feeling betrayed by a body that was suddenly doing things he'd worked so hard to stop. His husband held him and reminded him: this was temporary, purposeful, chosen. But that didn't make it easy.

If you're a transgender man considering pregnancy, you need specific information about how testosterone affects fertility, what stopping it involves, managing dysphoria during conception and pregnancy, and finding providers who actually understand trans pregnancy. This chapter is your guide.

6.1 Testosterone and Fertility

Testosterone suppresses ovulation in most transgender men, but it doesn't eliminate the capacity for pregnancy and doesn't permanently damage fertility in most cases.

How testosterone affects reproductive function: Testosterone therapy causes the following changes relevant to fertility:

- Stops menstruation in most users within 2-6 months
- Suppresses ovulation (but not in everyone—breakthrough ovulation can occur)
- Thickens cervical mucus

- Reduces endometrial lining thickness
- May cause some atrophy of reproductive organs with long-term use

But here's what testosterone doesn't do: it doesn't destroy eggs, doesn't prevent fertility restoration when stopped, and doesn't make pregnancy impossible if you're having sex that could result in conception (Light et al., 2014).

Pregnancy while on testosterone: It's possible to become pregnant while taking testosterone, particularly in early months of therapy before ovulation fully suppresses. Testosterone is not birth control. If you're having sex that could result in pregnancy and don't want to become pregnant, use contraception even while on testosterone.

If you discover you're pregnant while on testosterone, stop immediately and seek prenatal care. Limited research exists on testosterone exposure in early pregnancy, but available evidence suggests that stopping testosterone promptly doesn't typically cause problems (Light et al., 2014).

Fertility after testosterone: Most transgender men who stop testosterone eventually regain fertility. The timeline varies:

- Some resume ovulation within 1-2 months
- Most resume within 3-6 months
- Some take 6-12 months or longer
- A small percentage have difficulty resuming regular cycles

Longer duration of testosterone use doesn't necessarily mean longer recovery time. Some people who've been on testosterone for ten years resume cycling quickly. Others who've been on it for one year take many months. Individual variation is significant.

6.2 Stopping Testosterone

If you've decided to pursue pregnancy, you'll need to stop testosterone. This involves physical changes and often significant dysphoria.

When to stop: Most providers recommend stopping testosterone at least 2-3 months before actively trying to conceive. This allows time for your cycle to return and for residual testosterone to clear your system. Some people conceive successfully sooner if they resume ovulation quickly.

Physical changes to expect:

- Return of menstruation (typically within 1-6 months)
- Breast tissue may become slightly more prominent
- Fat redistribution toward hips and thighs over time
- Reduction in muscle mass (gradual)
- Skin may become less oily
- Libido changes (varies by person)
- Energy level changes

Your voice won't change back. Facial hair won't disappear. Body hair may thin slightly but remains. Bottom growth (clitoral enlargement) is permanent. Many masculinizing effects of testosterone persist even after stopping.

Cycle monitoring: Track when your period returns and what your cycles look like. Use ovulation tracking methods from Chapter 4.0 to identify when you're ovulating. Some transgender men have irregular cycles initially as their bodies adjust.

If your period doesn't return within six months of stopping testosterone, consult a healthcare provider. You might need hormonal intervention to restart cycling.

6.3 Dysphoria Management

Stopping testosterone and becoming pregnant often trigger significant dysphoria. Planning for this ahead of time helps.

Common dysphoria triggers during conception phase:

- Menstruation returning
- Needing to use menstrual products
- Body changes toward more feminine fat distribution
- Breast tissue changes
- Medical providers using feminine language or treating you as a woman
- Fertility tracking involving attention to cervical mucus, vaginal changes, etc.
- Vulnerability and loss of control

Coping strategies:

Reframe the experience: Some transgender men find it helpful to view pregnancy as an intensely masculine experience—using their male body's capacity to create life. Others frame it as a temporary medical condition they're undergoing to achieve a goal. Find the mental framework that works for you.

Maintain other masculine markers: Continue to present however feels authentic. Bind if you're not actively trying to conceive or in early pregnancy (stop binding once pregnant). Use masculine pronouns, name, and identity consistently. Your pregnancy doesn't make you less male.

Therapy support: Work with a therapist who understands transgender identities and reproductive experiences. Having professional support for dysphoria management matters.

Community connection: Connect with other transgender men who've been through pregnancy. Online communities exist specifically for trans pregnancy. You're not alone in this experience, even though it feels rare.

Communicate needs clearly: Tell your partner, care providers, and support people what language you need, what touches feel okay, what help you want. Don't assume people know. Give explicit guidance.

Plan for resuming testosterone: Knowing you can restart testosterone after pregnancy and chest-feeding (if applicable) provides a light at the end of the tunnel. This is temporary.

6.4 Conception Methods

Transgender men use the same conception methods as cisgender women—at-home insemination, IUI, or IVF. The methods work the same way biologically.

At-home insemination: Perfectly viable if you have regular cycles after stopping testosterone, no fertility issues, and access to sperm (known donor or purchased from sperm bank). Follow the process from section 5.3 in Chapter 5.0.

Track ovulation, time insemination attempts for your fertile window, use sterile techniques, and plan for multiple attempts over several cycles.

Clinical IUI: Works well for transgender men who want medical support and monitoring. IUI provides precise timing through trigger shots and monitoring, potentially improving success rates.

Some transgender men appreciate IUI because it minimizes dysphoric physical interactions—the medical procedure feels more clinical and less intimate than at-home methods.

IVF: Recommended if you have fertility challenges, have tried multiple cycles unsuccessfully, or want to complete your family building before resuming testosterone long-term. IVF allows you to retrieve and fertilize eggs, create embryos, transfer some for immediate pregnancy, and freeze others for future children. This means you can stop testosterone once, complete one retrieval, and potentially have multiple children without needing to stop testosterone again.

Partner involvement: If you have a partner with a uterus who could carry, you might consider providing eggs for your partner to carry (the inverse of reciprocal IVF for lesbian couples). This means you stop testosterone long enough for egg retrieval but don't have to experience pregnancy yourself. Your partner carries your biological child.

6.5 Finding Trans Competent Providers

Not all fertility specialists or midwives understand transgender pregnancy. Finding providers who won't treat you like a confused woman matters enormously for your mental health and quality of care.

What to look for in providers:

- Immediate use of correct pronouns and name
- Experience with transgender pregnancy (ask how many trans patients they've worked with)
- Comfortable with male pregnant people (not acting like it's shocking or weird)
- Knowledge about testosterone's effects on fertility and pregnancy
- Willingness to use your preferred language for anatomy
- Ability to handle insurance issues around gender markers
- Advocacy for you with hospital systems

Questions to ask potential providers:

- Have you cared for transgender men during pregnancy?
- How do you document gender in your systems when it doesn't match reproductive capacity?
- How do you prepare hospital staff for transgender patients during labor?
- Are you comfortable with me using male pronouns and being called a father?
- What's your understanding of how testosterone affects fertility and pregnancy?

- Can you provide references from other transgender clients?

Red flags:

- Repeated pronoun mistakes or use of feminine language after correction
- Treating your pregnancy as something strange or unusual
- Lack of knowledge about testosterone and pregnancy
- Discomfort with your identity
- Focusing excessively on your transgender status rather than your pregnancy

6.6 Pregnancy After Conception

Once you're pregnant, you'll deal with pregnancy-specific challenges covered in Chapter 13.0 (trans pregnancy experiences). But during the conception phase, prepare mentally for what's ahead:

Continuing dysphoria: Pregnancy makes your body more feminine-appearing. Breasts grow. Hips widen. Your shape becomes curvy. You'll be visibly pregnant and people will gender you female based on appearance. This triggers dysphoria for most transgender men.

Misgendering: Expect constant misgendering once pregnancy is visible. Strangers will call you "mom," "ma'am," and assume you're female. Even people who knew you as male might slip up. This is exhausting and distressing.

Medical interactions: You'll have frequent medical appointments throughout pregnancy. Every interaction is a chance for affirming care or for discrimination and erasure. Having good providers (from section 6.5) makes this manageable.

Physical changes: Pregnancy changes your body in ways testosterone had reversed—breasts, curves, softness. Remind yourself these changes are temporary and purposeful.

Mental health: Many transgender men struggle with prenatal mental health due to dysphoria, discrimination, and the difficulty of being pregnant while male. Line up therapeutic support before conception. Don't wait until you're in crisis.

6.7 Conception Timeline Example

Consider this composite timeline: Kai decided at age 28 to pursue pregnancy. He'd been on testosterone for five years. He and his cisgender male partner wanted children and chose for Kai to carry because surrogacy was financially out of reach.

Months 1-3: Kai stopped testosterone and began therapy focused on dysphoria management. His period returned at month two. He started tracking his cycles.

Months 4-6: Kai's cycles were irregular initially. He used ovulation predictor kits and began at-home insemination attempts. Three cycles of insemination with well-timed attempts. No pregnancy.

Months 7-9: Kai consulted with a trans-competent fertility specialist. Basic workup showed no fertility issues—he just needed more time. He continued at-home insemination for three more cycles.

Month 10: Pregnancy achieved on the sixth insemination attempt. Kai was simultaneously relieved and terrified. The pregnancy meant success but also nine more months of dysphoria and being off testosterone.

Pregnancy: Kai worked with a midwife experienced in trans pregnancy, attended transgender parent support groups online, continued therapy, and managed dysphoria with strong support systems. He gave birth at 39 weeks. His son was healthy.

Postpartum: Kai didn't chest-feed (he'd had top surgery before pregnancy and couldn't produce milk). He resumed testosterone at six weeks postpartum. Within months, he felt more like himself physically while adjusting to new parenthood.

His advice to other transgender men: "It's harder than you think it'll be, but also more worth it than you can imagine. You don't stop being a man because you're pregnant. You're just a man doing something most men can't do."

6.8 Special Considerations

Top surgery and pregnancy: If you've had top surgery, you can still become pregnant. Top surgery removes breast tissue, which means you likely can't chest-feed after pregnancy, but it doesn't affect fertility or pregnancy itself. Your chest might experience some soreness during pregnancy as hormones affect remaining tissue, but major changes are unlikely.

Bottom surgery and pregnancy: If you've had any bottom surgery (metoidioplasty or phalloplasty), you can't become pregnant through vaginal conception. The surgical changes eliminate the vaginal canal. You'd need to provide eggs for a partner or surrogate to carry.

Hysterectomy and pregnancy: If you've had a hysterectomy (uterus removal), you can't carry a pregnancy. You could potentially provide eggs for a partner or surrogate to carry if you still have ovaries, but carrying yourself isn't possible.

Fertility preservation: If you're not ready to pursue pregnancy now but want the option later, consider egg freezing before starting testosterone or during a pause in testosterone therapy. This preserves fertility if you're uncertain about future family plans. See section 2.6 in Chapter 2.0 for details.

6.9 Partner Support

If you have a partner involved in this conception process, they need guidance on how to support you.

What partners can do:

- Learn about transgender pregnancy and dysphoria
- Use correct pronouns and language consistently, especially in medical settings
- Advocate with providers on your behalf
- Check in about dysphoria without making assumptions
- Provide physical and emotional support throughout
- Remind you that you're still male, still you, even while pregnant
- Take over tasks that trigger dysphoria if possible
- Celebrate your strength in doing this difficult thing

What partners should avoid:

- Using feminine language about your body or pregnancy
- Telling you to "just get through it" without acknowledging difficulty
- Minimizing dysphoria as not that bad
- Making the pregnancy all about their experience and excitement
- Failing to advocate when you're misgendered by others
- Assuming you'll enjoy pregnancy experiences that cisgender women might enjoy

6.10 Moving Forward

Transgender men can and do conceive and carry healthy pregnancies successfully. It requires stopping testosterone, managing dysphoria, finding competent providers, and maintaining strong support systems. The process is challenging, but many transgender men report that it's worth it to have biological children.

In Chapter 7.0, we'll cover surrogacy for gay male couples. Chapter 8.0 discusses alternative family configurations. Chapter 9.0 addresses fertility challenges and emotional aspects when conception takes time.

For transgender men specifically, Chapter 13.0 (in Part Three) provides detailed guidance on pregnancy experiences, and Chapter 20.0 covers labor and birth considerations.

6.11 Core Concepts

Testosterone suppresses but doesn't eliminate fertility in most transgender men. Stopping testosterone allows fertility to return, usually within 3-6 months. Conception methods are the same as for cisgender women. Dysphoria management requires planning, support, and reframing strategies. Finding trans-competent providers who respect your male identity while providing prenatal care is essential.

Pregnancy as a transgender man is possible and increasingly common. You're not alone in this experience, even though it feels rare. Connect with community, line up support, and trust that you can do this difficult, worthwhile thing.

Chapter 7.0: Surrogacy for Gay Couples

David and Carlos started researching surrogacy the way most people research buying cars—spreadsheets, comparison charts, budgets. They quickly discovered that nothing about surrogacy resembles buying cars. They were building a relationship with a woman who would carry their child. They were navigating complex legal systems. They were facing costs that made them question everything.

Three years later, when their daughter was born, they both understood: surrogacy is complicated, expensive, emotionally intense, and for many gay male couples, the only path to biological parenthood. If this is your path, you need comprehensive information about how surrogacy works, what it costs, how to find surrogates and agencies, and how to build connection with your child when you're not the one pregnant.

7.1 Gestational Surrogacy Overview

Gestational surrogacy means a surrogate (also called a gestational carrier) carries a pregnancy created through IVF using eggs from an egg donor and sperm from one or both intended fathers. The surrogate has no genetic connection to the baby—she's carrying your biological child, not hers.

This differs from **traditional surrogacy** where a surrogate's own eggs are used, making her genetically related to the child. Traditional surrogacy is legally riskier and ethically complicated. Most agencies and attorneys work exclusively with gestational surrogacy now.

The basic process:

1. Select egg donor (anonymous or known)
2. Find and match with a surrogate
3. Complete legal contracts
4. IVF cycle with egg donor and intended father's sperm
5. Embryo transfer to surrogate
6. Surrogate carries pregnancy
7. Birth and custody transfer to intended parents

This process takes 12-24 months from starting to search for a surrogate through birth, and costs $100,000-$200,000 depending on location and specifics.

7.2 The Financial Reality

Let's be direct about costs because this information is often hard to find. Surrogacy is expensive. Most middle-class families can't afford it without loans, savings, or significant financial planning.

Cost breakdown:

- **Surrogate compensation**: $30,000-$60,000 for base compensation (varies by location, experience, state)
- **Surrogate expenses**: $15,000-$30,000 for medical expenses, maternity clothes, travel, lost wages if on bed rest, childcare for surrogate's children during appointments
- **Agency fees**: $20,000-$40,000 if using an agency to match with surrogate
- **IVF costs**: $15,000-$25,000 per cycle including egg donor fees, medications, procedures, embryo creation
- **Legal fees**: $10,000-$20,000 for contracts, parentage orders, surrogate's legal representation
- **Insurance**: $10,000-$30,000 for surrogacy insurance or to cover surrogate's medical costs if her insurance excludes surrogacy
- **Miscellaneous**: $5,000-$10,000 for screening, background checks, travel, additional contingencies

Total estimated costs: $100,000-$150,000 for standard arrangements without complications. Costs increase if multiple IVF cycles are needed, if complications arise during pregnancy, or if you're in high-cost states like California or New York.

This is prohibitive for many families. Some financing options exist: surrogacy-specific loans from companies like New Life Fertility Finance, home equity loans, retirement account loans, grants from LGBTQ+ family organizations (limited availability), employer benefits (increasingly available at LGBTQ+-friendly companies).

Plan realistically. Understand that you might need to save for years before pursuing surrogacy, or that you might need to explore international surrogacy in countries with lower costs (though this brings additional legal complexities).

7.3 Finding a Surrogate

You can find surrogates independently or through agencies. Each approach has benefits and complications.

Using a surrogacy agency:

Benefits:

- Agencies screen surrogates medically and psychologically
- Agencies handle matching based on your preferences
- They coordinate medical, legal, and logistical details
- They provide support throughout the process
- They ensure surrogates meet criteria (age, previous successful pregnancies, medical health, etc.)

Drawbacks:

- Expensive ($20,000-$40,000 in agency fees)
- Less control over surrogate selection
- Agencies vary in quality and LGBTQ+ affirmation

Finding surrogates independently:

Benefits:

- Save agency fees
- More control over selection
- Direct relationship with surrogate
- Can be faster if you already have someone in mind

Drawbacks:

- You're responsible for screening, contracts, coordination
- More legal complexity
- Risk of matching with someone unsuitable
- Harder to find surrogates without agency databases

Who can be a surrogate:

Most programs require surrogates to meet specific criteria:

- Age 21-40 (most agencies prefer 21-37)
- At least one previous successful pregnancy and delivery
- Currently raising at least one of their children (proves they understand parenthood)
- Healthy BMI (typically 19-32)
- Non-smoker, no drug use
- Stable living situation
- Psychological health screening
- Medical screening for uterine health and previous pregnancy complications
- US citizen or legal resident (for domestic surrogacy)

Where to find surrogates:

If going independently, you might find surrogates through:

- Personal networks (friends, relatives, acquaintances who volunteer)

- Online matching sites (SurrogateWeb, Surrogate.com)
- Social media groups for surrogacy
- Word of mouth in LGBTQ+ communities

If using agencies, research thoroughly: check reviews, ask for references from other gay couples, verify LGBTQ+ competency, understand their screening processes and matching criteria.

7.4 The Matching Process

Matching with a surrogate involves both parties determining compatibility—you're essentially choosing someone to have a profound, intimate relationship with for the next year.

What surrogates consider: Surrogates evaluate intended parents based on:

- Personality compatibility
- Communication style
- Relationship stability
- Parenting philosophy
- Level of involvement they want during pregnancy
- Financial stability
- How they'll support the surrogate

What you should consider: Evaluate potential surrogates based on:

- Previous pregnancy history (uncomplicated pregnancies are ideal)
- Lifestyle and health habits
- Communication preferences
- Personality fit
- Willingness to follow medical protocols
- Her family's support for surrogacy
- Her motivation for being a surrogate
- Compatibility on key issues (selective reduction, pregnancy termination for medical reasons, etc.)

The matching meeting: Most matches involve meeting (in person or virtually) to discuss:

- Expectations throughout pregnancy
- Communication frequency and methods
- Involvement during pregnancy (appointments, ultrasounds, birth)
- Boundaries and preferences
- Practical logistics
- Legal and financial details

Both parties should leave matching meetings feeling positive and comfortable. If something feels off, don't proceed just because you're anxious to move forward. The relationship matters.

7.5 Legal Framework

Surrogacy laws vary dramatically by state. Some states are very surrogacy-friendly. Others make surrogacy difficult or legally risky. Some ban commercial surrogacy entirely.

Surrogacy-friendly states: California, Connecticut, Delaware, Nevada, New Hampshire, Washington, and several others allow surrogacy with straightforward legal processes for establishing parental rights (Caplan & Levine, 2017).

Complicated or restrictive states: Michigan, Louisiana, Nebraska ban or severely restrict surrogacy. New York only recently legalized compensated surrogacy. Some states have uncertain or untested legal frameworks.

Why state matters: You need enforceable contracts and clear processes for establishing legal parentage. In surrogacy-friendly states, you can often obtain pre-birth orders that establish you as legal parents before the baby is born. In other states, you might need adoption proceedings after birth.

Work with attorneys specializing in reproductive law and surrogacy, particularly those familiar with LGBTQ+ family building. Never proceed without proper legal representation for both you and your surrogate.

What surrogacy contracts cover:

- Surrogate compensation and expenses
- Medical decisions during pregnancy
- Intended parents' involvement during pregnancy and birth
- What happens if pregnancy doesn't occur or ends in miscarriage
- Plans for complications (multiples, medical problems, etc.)
- Termination decisions if medical issues arise
- Post-birth contact expectations
- Custody transfer process
- Dispute resolution

Both parties need independent legal counsel. You pay for your attorney and the surrogate's attorney. This ensures the surrogate understands her rights and that contracts are enforceable.

7.6 The IVF Process

Creating embryos for surrogacy involves IVF using an egg donor's eggs and your sperm.

Egg donor selection: Similar to sperm donor selection for lesbian couples (covered in section 5.8), you'll review donor profiles choosing based on physical characteristics, intelligence, health history, ethnicity, and other factors. Some people use known egg donors (relatives or friends). Others use anonymous donors from agencies.

Egg donor fees range from $5,000-$15,000 depending on donor desirability and agency fees.

The IVF cycle:

1. Egg donor takes stimulation medications for 8-14 days
2. Egg retrieval when eggs are mature
3. Your sperm (or both partners' sperm mixed) fertilizes eggs in lab
4. Embryos develop for 5-6 days to blastocyst stage
5. Embryos can be genetically tested (PGT-A testing) to check for chromosomal abnormalities
6. One embryo is transferred to surrogate's uterus
7. Remaining embryos are frozen for future use

Whose sperm: If both partners want biological connection, some couples mix sperm so biological paternity is unknown until birth or remains unknown forever. Others designate one partner as biological father for the first child and alternate for subsequent children. Some couples use one partner's sperm exclusively. There's no right answer—just the answer that fits your relationship.

Success rates: IVF success rates depend on egg donor age (younger donors have better outcomes). With donors under 30, success rates per embryo transfer are approximately 60-70% (Society for Assisted Reproductive Technology, 2022). Most couples achieve pregnancy within 1-2 embryo transfer attempts.

7.7 Supporting Your Surrogate

Your surrogate is doing something profound for your family. Supporting her well matters ethically and practically.

During pregnancy:

- Maintain regular communication (texts, calls, video chats—whatever frequency you've agreed on)
- Attend medical appointments if she's comfortable with that
- Send care packages or small gifts
- Check in about how she's feeling physically and emotionally
- Respect her boundaries while showing appreciation
- Provide the financial support you've contracted for promptly
- Be available for questions or concerns

Practical support:

- Cover all agreed-upon expenses quickly
- Help coordinate medical appointments or provide transportation if needed
- Provide childcare funds if she needs care for her kids during appointments
- Send meal delivery or practical help if she's on bed rest
- Be responsive to texts and calls

Emotional boundaries: Your surrogate is carrying your baby, but she's not your employee. She's a person doing something extraordinary who deserves respect, gratitude, and appropriate boundaries. Don't treat her as a commodity. Don't micromanage her life. Don't demand excessive updates.

Most surrogate-intended parent relationships develop into genuine friendships based on mutual respect and shared experience.

7.8 Building Connection During Pregnancy

One challenge for intended fathers using surrogacy: you can't feel the baby move, attend prenatal appointments as the patient, or experience physical connection to your growing child. Building connection requires intention.

Ways to connect:

- Attend ultrasound appointments (with surrogate's permission)
- Ask surrogate to send photos or videos of her belly
- Talk or sing to the baby during video calls with surrogate
- Create playlist for baby and have surrogate play it
- Read pregnancy books and follow baby's development week by week
- Prepare nursery and baby items
- Attend prenatal classes

- Build connection with the idea of your child even without physical connection
- Journal about your feelings and thoughts for the baby

Partner involvement: Both partners should stay actively involved if you're a couple. Don't let one partner become more connected because he provided sperm or takes point on communication with the surrogate. Share appointments, updates, preparations, and emotional experience.

7.9 Birth and Postpartum

When birth approaches, you'll need plans for being present, taking custody, and bonding with your newborn.

Birth presence: Most surrogates welcome intended parents at the birth, but discuss this explicitly. Where will you be during labor? In the delivery room? Who cuts the cord? Can you do skin-to-skin immediately?

Hospital policies: Work with the hospital in advance to ensure:

- You're allowed in the delivery room (most hospitals allow intended parents now)
- You can take custody of the baby immediately
- Birth certificates reflect correct parentage
- You can room with the baby
- Staff understand the surrogacy arrangement

Immediate postpartum: You'll take custody of your baby immediately after birth. The surrogate typically spends minimal time with the baby—this isn't her child; she's completed her role. You start parenting immediately.

Feeding: You'll formula-feed unless you've arranged for donor milk or induced lactation (rare but possible in some situations). Prepare bottles, formula, and feeding supplies in advance.

Post-birth relationship: Discuss expectations for post-birth contact before birth. Some surrogates and intended parents maintain close friendships. Others prefer minimal contact after delivery. Neither approach is wrong—just different preferences.

7.10 Real World Example

Consider Carlos and David's journey (composite): They spent two years saving $120,000 for surrogacy. They used an agency in California and matched with Emma, a 28-year-old mother of two who'd been a surrogate once before. Carlos provided sperm. They used an anonymous egg donor who looked similar to David's sister.

The first IVF cycle created seven embryos. The first transfer worked. Emma had an uncomplicated pregnancy. Carlos and David attended all major ultrasounds via video (they lived across the country from Emma). They texted weekly and video-called monthly.

When Emma went into labor, they flew to California. They were in the delivery room when their daughter was born. Carlos cut the cord. They did immediate skin-to-skin. Emma held the baby briefly to say goodbye and congratulations, then returned home to her family.

Carlos and David spent three days in the hospital learning infant care, then brought their daughter home. Emma texted occasionally to check how they were doing. They sent photos and updates. The relationship was warm but bounded.

Their advice: "It's expensive and complicated, but worth every penny and every frustration. Our daughter is perfect. Emma gave us the greatest gift imaginable."

7.11 Essential Considerations

Surrogacy for gay male couples requires:

- Significant financial resources ($100,000-$200,000)
- 12-24 months from start to birth

- Legal representation in surrogacy-friendly states
- Careful surrogate screening and matching
- IVF with egg donor
- Strong support and communication with surrogate
- Planning for birth and immediate postpartum
- Preparation for formula feeding and infant care without pregnancy experience

Despite challenges, many gay male couples report that surrogacy, though expensive and complex, allows them to become biological parents in a way that feels deeply meaningful.

Chapter 8.0: Alternative Family Configurations

When Riley, Jordan, and Alex decided to have a baby together, they hit an immediate problem: there was no guidebook. Three-parent families exist in LGBTQ+ communities, but resources assume two parents—one biological, one not, or two biological parents in straight relationships, or two moms, or two dads. Not three parents who all wanted equal involvement and legal recognition.

They figured it out anyway. Riley carried. Jordan provided sperm. Alex co-parented from day one. Their son has three parents who share custody, decisions, and all the work. It's not conventional, but it works beautifully for them.

This chapter covers alternative family configurations that don't fit the two-parent model: polyamorous families, co-parenting arrangements between non-romantic partners, single LGBTQ+ parents by choice, and families involving chosen family or extended networks. If your family doesn't fit standard molds, this is your chapter.

8.1 Co-Parenting Arrangements

Co-parenting means people who aren't romantic partners choose to have and raise children together. This happens across sexual orientations but is particularly common in LGBTQ+ communities where people might want children but not romantic partnerships, or want to parent with friends rather than partners.

Why co-parenting:

- Single people who want children but don't have partners

- Friends who want to parent together without romantic involvement
- Gay men and lesbian women partnering to have biological children they co-parent
- People prioritizing parenting compatibility over romantic attraction

Successful co-parenting requires:

Clear agreements upfront: Before conception, discuss and ideally document:

- Legal parentage (who will be legal parents?)
- Custody and living arrangements (will child live with one parent primarily, or split time?)
- Decision-making authority (medical, educational, religious, etc.)
- Financial responsibilities (who pays for what?)
- Involvement of co-parents' future romantic partners
- What happens if co-parents move to different cities
- Dispute resolution if you disagree on major issues

Legal documentation: Work with attorneys to create co-parenting agreements that outline rights, responsibilities, and expectations. These aren't always legally enforceable like custody orders in divorces, but they provide frameworks and can inform court decisions if disputes arise.

Realistic expectations: Co-parenting without romantic partnership is different from parenting with a romantic partner. You won't necessarily live together. You'll need explicit communication about everything since you can't assume shared understanding. You'll need mechanisms for resolving disagreements.

Case example (composite): Marcus (a gay man) and Jennifer (a lesbian woman) became close friends in college. Both wanted children but hadn't found long-term romantic partners by their mid-30s. They decided to co-parent together.

Jennifer carried their child using Marcus's sperm. They lived in different apartments in the same city. Their daughter spent three days with Marcus, four days with Jennifer, with flexible adjustments based on work and life demands. They made all major decisions together, splitting costs equally.

When Jennifer later partnered with another woman, her girlfriend became an additional supportive adult in their daughter's life, but Jennifer and Marcus remained the legal parents with equal authority.

It worked because they had clear agreements, genuine respect for each other, compatible parenting values, and willingness to communicate constantly.

8.2 Polyamorous Families

Polyamorous families—where more than two adults are in committed romantic relationships—sometimes include children. Legal and social systems struggle with this reality, but these families exist and function.

Configurations vary:

- Three adults in a relationship (a "triad") deciding to have children together
- Four or more adults in various relationship configurations (a "quad" or larger polycule)
- "Vee" relationships where one person has two partners who aren't romantically involved with each other
- More complex networks

Pregnancy in polyamorous families:

Who carries? If multiple people have uteruses, deciding who carries involves the same considerations as lesbian couples (section 5.1 in Chapter 5.0) plus navigating more than two people's input.

Who provides genetics? If multiple people could provide sperm or eggs, families navigate complex questions about biological connection. Some mix sperm to create uncertainty. Some intentionally use specific biological parents. Some do sequential children with different biological parents.

How many legal parents? This is where polyamorous families hit legal walls. Most states only allow two legal parents maximum. A few jurisdictions recognize three parents in specific circumstances. This creates vulnerability—some parents have no legal relationship to children they're actively parenting.

Legal strategies for polyamorous families:

- Two parents establish legal parentage through birth certificates or adoption
- Non-legal parents establish rights through:
    - Powers of attorney for medical and educational decisions
    - Guardianship arrangements
    - De facto parent status (recognition of parent-like relationships through years of involvement)
    - Wills specifying custody preferences if legal parents die
    - Co-parenting agreements (similar to section 8.1) outlining roles and responsibilities

Challenges:

- Lack of legal recognition for all parents creates insecurity
- Healthcare systems and schools struggle with more than two parents
- Extended family might not understand or accept family structure
- Moving to different states might change legal landscape

Benefits:

- More adults sharing parenting work and costs
- Children have multiple attachment figures
- Built-in support systems
- Modeling of ethical non-monogamy for children

Consider a composite example: Riley, Jordan, and Alex (mentioned in the chapter opening) created a three-parent family. Riley carried using Jordan's sperm. Alex had no biological connection but was equally involved from conception planning forward.

Legally, Riley and Jordan are the recognized parents. Alex has power of attorney for medical and educational decisions, and their co-parenting agreement specifies his equal role. Their son knows all three as parents and spends time in both households (Riley and Alex live together; Jordan lives nearby).

It's unconventional, but their son is loved, secure, and thriving. The legal complications are real—they consulted attorneys extensively and continue updating documents as laws change.

8.3 Single LGBTQ Parents

Many LGBTQ+ people choose single parenthood—no partner, no co-parent, just them and their child. This is increasingly common and completely valid, but it requires specific planning.

Conception options for single LGBTQ+ parents:

For people with uteruses: Use donor sperm (anonymous or known) for at-home insemination, IUI, or IVF. Process is identical to lesbian couples (Chapter 5.0) except you're making all decisions alone and providing all support yourself.

For people with testes: Use surrogacy (Chapter 7.0) plus egg donor. This is more expensive and complex, but single gay men and transgender women successfully build families this way.

Why single parenthood by choice:

- Not finding appropriate co-parent or romantic partner
- Preferring independence in parenting decisions
- Biological clock concerns making it impractical to wait for partners
- Previous relationship trauma making partnership difficult
- Simply wanting to parent alone

Challenges of single LGBTQ+ parenthood:

- All costs fall on one person
- No built-in co-parent to share physical and emotional work
- Less time for self-care and personal needs
- Potentially less support from biological family if they're unsupportive of LGBTQ+ identity
- Need to build intentional support networks

Strategies for success:

- Build strong support networks before conception (friends, chosen family, community)
- Save more money than couples need (you're covering everything alone)
- Plan for childcare and backup care
- Connect with single parent communities for support
- Consider living near family or friends who can help
- Line up practical help for postpartum period
- Be realistic about what single parenthood involves

Legal considerations: Single parents have clear legal parentage—you're the only parent unless you use a known donor without proper legal agreements. Ensure you have wills specifying guardianship if something happens to you, since no automatic second parent exists.

8.4 Chosen Family Involvement

Many LGBTQ+ people have created families of choice—close friends who function as family. These relationships can be incorporated into family building in various ways.

Ways chosen family can be involved:

- Close friends serving as donors (sperm donors, egg donors, surrogates)
- Friends providing intensive support during pregnancy, birth, and postpartum
- "Aunties," "uncles," or other honorary family roles for chosen family members
- Guardianship arrangements naming chosen family as guardians if parents die
- Including chosen family in major decisions and celebrations

Importance of chosen family for LGBTQ+ parents: Biological families sometimes reject LGBTQ+ people or don't support their family building. Chosen family fills these gaps, providing emotional support, practical help, and celebrating milestones that biological families might ignore or oppose.

Making expectations clear: If chosen family will be heavily involved, discuss expectations before conception:

- What role will they play?
- What help will you ask for?
- What boundaries exist?
- How permanent is this involvement?

Don't assume chosen family automatically wants intensive involvement. Ask explicitly and respect their capacity.

8.5 Multi-Parent Legal Recognition

A handful of jurisdictions now recognize more than two legal parents in specific circumstances. This is evolving legal territory.

Where it's possible: California, Delaware, Maine, Vermont, and Washington have laws or court precedents allowing three or more legal parents when it serves the child's best interest. Requirements and processes vary by state.

When it's granted: Courts typically recognize additional parents when:

- Child has been raised by more than two adults functioning as parents
- All adults agree to multi-parent recognition
- It's in the child's best interest to maintain all parent-child relationships
- Biological and non-biological parents all seek recognition

Limitations: Even in states allowing multi-parent recognition, it's not automatic. It requires legal processes, often including all parties going to court to establish parentage. And it only applies to the state granting it—other states might not recognize the legal arrangement.

Importance: For polyamorous families and co-parenting arrangements with more than two adults, legal recognition of all parents provides security. Everyone has legal rights to make decisions, consent to medical care, and maintain custody.

8.6 Practical Realities

Alternative family configurations require additional planning and flexibility compared to two-parent families because systems aren't designed for you.

School forms: They'll ask for "Mother" and "Father" or "Parent 1" and "Parent 2." What do you do with three parents? Or one parent? Or co-parents who aren't partners?

Work with schools proactively: explain your family structure, provide all parents' contact information, clarify who has authority to make decisions and pick up the child. Good schools accommodate. Less flexible schools create friction.

Medical care: Pediatricians need to know who can consent to treatment, who should receive medical information, and who to contact in emergencies. Provide clear documentation of legal relationships and medical powers of attorney for non-legal parents.

Social situations: People will ask about your family structure. Kids will ask your kids. Nosy neighbors will make assumptions. You need responses ready:

"She has three parents who all love and care for her."

"I'm a single parent by choice, and I have amazing friends who help."

"His parents aren't together romantically, but we co-parent together."

Whatever explanation feels authentic and age-appropriate.

8.7 Your Path Forward

If your family configuration doesn't fit standard models, you'll need to:

1. **Get legal guidance early**: Work with attorneys specializing in LGBTQ+ family law and alternative family structures to protect everyone's rights.
2. **Create explicit agreements**: Document expectations, responsibilities, and decision-making processes.
3. **Build support networks**: Especially crucial if you're single parenting or if biological families aren't supportive.
4. **Prepare for systems that don't fit**: Schools, medical offices, legal documents—they'll assume two parents or one parent. You'll need to explain and advocate repeatedly.
5. **Connect with community**: Other people in alternative family configurations exist. Finding them reduces isolation and provides practical wisdom.

Alternative families work. They require more intentionality and more advocacy, but children thrive when they're loved and supported by committed adults, regardless of whether those adults fit conventional definitions of family.

8.8 Core Principles

Co-parenting arrangements between non-romantic partners succeed with clear agreements, legal documentation, and commitment to communication. Polyamorous families navigate legal limitations by strategically establishing parentage for two adults and using legal tools (powers of attorney, guardianship, co-parenting agreements) for additional parents. Single LGBTQ+ parents build strong support networks and plan financially for sole responsibility. Chosen family fills gaps left by unsupportive biological families.

All alternative family configurations require advocacy because systems assume two-parent, romantically-involved structures. But these families exist, function well, and raise healthy, happy children.

Chapter 9.0: When Conception Takes Time

Elena started crying in the bathroom when she saw blood for the sixth time. Six cycles. Six negative pregnancy tests. She and Jasmine had done everything right—perfect timing, quality sperm, no known fertility issues. But month after month, nothing.

They felt alone until they found online forums full of other lesbian couples saying the same thing: "We thought it would be easy." "Everyone said we're young and healthy." "We've spent $8,000 and still no baby." Turns out, conception taking time is common even for people without fertility problems. But when you're paying for every attempt and watching your savings drain away, those statistics feel meaningless.

This chapter addresses what happens when conception takes longer than expected: the emotional toll, when to seek fertility support, how LGBTQ+ fertility testing differs from straight couple testing, dealing with secondary infertility, knowing when to stop trying, and considering alternatives like adoption or fostering. If you've been trying for a while with no success, this is for you.

9.1 The Emotional Toll

Straight couples who can accidentally conceive don't understand what it's like to plan, pay for, and wait for each conception attempt. LGBTQ+ people trying to conceive experience unique emotional challenges.

The financial stress: Every cycle costs money. Sperm costs $500-$1,000 per vial. IUI adds $300-$1,000 per cycle. IVF costs $12,000-$25,000. Failed attempts mean money gone with nothing to show for it. You watch your savings disappear while friends get pregnant accidentally. The financial pressure adds to emotional stress.

The isolation: Most LGBTQ+ people don't have large communities of other queer families to normalize the struggle. Your straight friends got pregnant quickly (or at least it seems that way). Your LGBTQ+ friends might not have kids yet. You feel alone.

The unfairness: It's not fair that straight people can conceive for free while you're paying thousands. It's not fair that you have to plan every detail while others just "see what happens." It's not fair that your body works fine but you still need medical intervention because of who you love. Grief about this unfairness is legitimate.

The uncertainty: You don't know if the next cycle will work or if you'll need 20 cycles. You don't know if something is wrong or if you're just unlucky. The uncertainty makes planning impossible and creates constant anxiety.

Relationship strain: Unsuccessful conception attempts strain relationships. Partners might have different risk tolerances for how much money to spend or how many attempts to try. Partners might blame themselves or each other. The stress affects intimacy, communication, and general happiness.

For transgender men specifically: Every failed cycle means more time off testosterone, more dysphoria, more delay before you can resume medical transition. The extended timeline compounds difficulty.

9.2 When Normal Becomes Concerning

How long is too long to keep trying before seeking fertility evaluation?

Standard advice for straight couples: Try for 12 months (if under 35) or six months (if over 35) before seeking evaluation. This assumes regular unprotected intercourse.

Modified advice for LGBTQ+ families: Consider evaluation after:

- Six cycles of well-timed attempts if under 35
- Three to four cycles if over 35
- Immediately if you have known risk factors (irregular cycles, PCOS, endometriosis, previous pelvic infections, previous fertility issues)

Why earlier? Because you're paying for each attempt. Because each cycle involves emotional energy. Because if something is preventing conception, you want to know sooner rather than later.

Success rate expectations: For fertile people under 35 with perfectly timed attempts, each cycle has about 15-20% success rate (Gnoth et al., 2003). This means 80-85% of cycles fail even with perfect timing and no fertility issues. After six cycles, about 60% of fertile people will have conceived. After 12 cycles, about 85%.

If you're not pregnant after six well-timed attempts and you're under 35, you're not necessarily infertile—you might just be in the unlucky 40%. But evaluation makes sense to rule out problems.

9.3 Fertility Testing for LGBTQ People

Fertility workup for LGBTQ+ people is similar to testing for straight couples but requires some modifications.

Standard fertility testing includes:

For people with uteruses:

- Hormone testing (FSH, LH, estradiol, AMH, thyroid hormones, prolactin)
- Ovarian reserve testing to assess egg quantity and quality
- Pelvic ultrasound to check uterus and ovaries
- HSG (hysterosalpingogram) to check if fallopian tubes are open

- Assessment of ovulation through tracking or progesterone blood tests
- Sometimes endometrial biopsy or additional testing

For people with testes:

- Semen analysis checking sperm count, motility, morphology
- Hormone testing if semen analysis is abnormal
- Physical exam

Modifications for LGBTQ+ testing:

For lesbian couples: Both partners might want fertility testing if you're deciding who should carry or if you're considering switching who tries after unsuccessful attempts.

For transgender men: Testing includes assessing how completely your cycle has returned after stopping testosterone and confirming ovulation is occurring. Some transgender men have irregular ovulation even after cycles return.

For gay male couples using surrogacy: Both partners can do semen analysis if planning to mix sperm, or just the partner who'll provide sperm can test.

Known donor testing: If using a known donor, he should complete semen analysis and STI testing before use. His sperm quality directly affects conception success.

9.4 Common Fertility Issues

Several conditions commonly prevent or delay conception.

Ovulation disorders: PCOS affects about 10% of women of reproductive age and causes irregular or absent ovulation (Azziz et al., 2016). If you don't ovulate regularly, timing insemination is difficult and success rates are lower. Treatment typically involves medications (letrozole or clomiphene) to induce ovulation.

Blocked fallopian tubes: Previous infections (particularly chlamydia or gonorrhea), endometriosis, or pelvic surgeries can block tubes, preventing sperm and egg from meeting. HSG testing identifies this. Treatment involves surgery to repair tubes or moving to IVF (which bypasses tubes).

Endometriosis: This condition, where uterine lining grows outside the uterus, affects about 10% of women and reduces fertility through inflammation, scarring, and anatomical distortion (Giudice, 2010). Treatment might include surgery, medications, or moving to IVF.

Uterine abnormalities: Fibroids, polyps, septate uterus, or other structural problems can prevent implantation. Surgical correction might be necessary.

Low ovarian reserve: As people age, egg quantity and quality decline. Testing (AMH, FSH, antral follicle count) assesses ovarian reserve. If reserve is low, IVF might be recommended sooner to maximize chances before it declines further.

Male factor infertility: If using a known donor, his sperm might have issues (low count, poor motility, abnormal morphology). This affects success with at-home insemination but might be overcome with IUI or IVF.

Unexplained infertility: Sometimes all testing comes back normal but pregnancy still doesn't occur. This is frustrating but common. Treatment often involves trying IUI or IVF even without a clear diagnosis.

9.5 Treatment Options

When fertility testing identifies issues or when conception hasn't happened after reasonable attempts, treatments can help.

Ovulation induction: Medications (letrozole, clomiphene) stimulate ovulation in people who don't ovulate regularly. Success rates improve significantly when ovulation is restored.

IUI (intrauterine insemination): Placing sperm directly in the uterus bypasses cervical mucus issues and places sperm closer to the egg. Success rates are 15-20% per cycle for people under 35 without fertility issues (Matorras et al., 2015).

IVF (in vitro fertilization): Creating embryos outside the body and transferring them to the uterus. IVF has the highest success rates per attempt (about 50% per transfer for people under 35) and is recommended for blocked tubes, severe male factor, failed IUI cycles, low ovarian reserve, or unexplained infertility after multiple attempts (Society for Assisted Reproductive Technology, 2022).

Surgery: Removing fibroids, repairing blocked tubes, treating endometriosis surgically. Surgery can restore fertility in some cases.

Deciding on treatment: Balance success rates, costs, invasiveness, and your specific diagnosis. Start with less invasive and cheaper options (ovulation induction, IUI) before moving to more intensive and expensive treatments (IVF) unless testing indicates you need to skip directly to IVF.

9.6 Secondary Infertility

Secondary infertility means difficulty conceiving after successfully having a previous biological child. This affects LGBTQ+ families just like straight families.

Why it happens: Fertility can change over time. Age, new medical conditions, changes in ovarian reserve, development of endometriosis or fibroids—any of these can reduce fertility even if you conceived easily before.

The unique pain: Secondary infertility feels different from primary infertility. You already have a child, so people assume you should feel grateful rather than grieving. But the desire for another child is legitimate, and the inability to conceive causes genuine pain.

Other parents sometimes say things like "At least you have one" or "Be grateful for what you have." These comments minimize your grief. Your desire for another child doesn't mean you're ungrateful for your existing child.

For lesbian couples: If one partner carried the first child easily and the other partner struggles conceiving the second child, jealousy and guilt can strain the relationship. The first partner might feel guilty for conceiving easily. The struggling partner might feel inadequate or resentful.

Moving forward: If you conceived easily the first time but struggle the second time, seek evaluation sooner. Something changed. Testing can identify what.

9.7 Deciding When to Stop

One of the hardest decisions in fertility journeys is knowing when to stop trying.

Factors in deciding:

Financial: How much money have you spent? How much more can you afford to spend? What's your limit?

Emotional: How much emotional capacity remains? Are you still hopeful, or has this become traumatic? How is it affecting your relationship, mental health, and quality of life?

Physical: For gestational parents, how many more cycles of hormones, procedures, and pregnancies can your body handle? For transgender men, how much longer can you tolerate being off testosterone?

Practical: How much more time can you dedicate to this? How does ongoing fertility treatment affect your work, other responsibilities, existing children?

Medical: What are your realistic chances given your age, diagnosis, and treatment history? Are doctors recommending stopping or continuing?

No universal timeline: Some people try for six months and decide to stop. Others try for five years. Neither is wrong. The right stopping point is the one where you've reached your emotional, financial, or physical limits.

Permission to stop: You're allowed to stop trying even if you haven't exhausted every possible option. You're allowed to decide that the cost (financial, emotional, physical) exceeds what you're willing to pay. Stopping isn't giving up—it's making a choice about what's sustainable for you.

Consider this composite example: Isabella and Jasmine tried for two years. Six cycles of IUI failed. Two IVF cycles failed. They'd spent $45,000. Isabella was emotionally exhausted and Jasmine was worried about her mental health. They decided to stop.

It felt like failure initially. But a year later, they'd fostered and then adopted a toddler. They loved their son and realized that conception wasn't the only path to parenthood. Stopping active fertility treatment freed them to pursue adoption, which turned out to be their path to family.

9.8 Alternatives to Biological Parenthood

If biological parenthood isn't happening or if you decide to stop pursuing it, other paths exist.

Adoption: Adopting children (infants or older children) through agencies or foster care. Many LGBTQ+ people build families through adoption. It's not a consolation prize—it's a different path to parenthood that's equally valid.

Foster care: Providing temporary or permanent homes to children who need them. Many LGBTQ+ people find fostering deeply meaningful. Some foster children eventually become available for adoption.

Child-free life: Deciding not to have children at all is a legitimate choice. Not everyone needs to be a parent. If fertility struggles reveal that actually you're okay not having children, that's valid.

Being part of children's lives without parenting: Auntie/uncle roles, godparents, mentoring, working with children professionally—these roles allow you to impact children's lives without being a parent.

9.9 Finding Support

Don't go through fertility struggles alone.

LGBTQ+ fertility support groups: Online communities exist specifically for LGBTQ+ people experiencing infertility. Search for "queer conception" groups, "lesbian TTC" (trying to conceive) groups, "trans pregnancy" forums. Talking to people who understand both the fertility struggles and the LGBTQ+ specific challenges helps.

General infertility support: Organizations like RESOLVE provide support groups, information, and advocacy for anyone experiencing infertility. While not LGBTQ+ specific, they can still help.

Therapy: Consider working with a therapist who specializes in infertility and LGBTQ+ issues. Processing grief, relationship strain, and decisions about whether to continue trying requires support.

Friends and chosen family: Don't isolate. Talk to supportive friends about what you're going through. Let people help.

9.10 Moving Forward

Conception taking longer than expected is emotionally devastating, financially draining, and isolating. You're not alone, you're not broken, and your feelings are valid.

Seek evaluation sooner than straight couples would because you're paying for attempts. Consider treatments that address identified problems. Make decisions about how long to continue based on your specific financial, emotional, and physical capacity. Know that alternatives exist if biological conception doesn't happen.

And remember: becoming a parent—however it happens—is what matters. The path there is just logistics.

9.11 Taking Stock

When conception takes time, remember:

- It's emotionally hard and your grief is valid
- Seek fertility evaluation after six cycles if under 35, three to four cycles if over 35
- Common fertility issues are treatable
- Treatment options range from simple (ovulation induction) to complex (IVF)
- You get to decide when to stop trying based on your limits
- Alternatives exist: adoption, fostering, child-free life
- Support helps: online communities, therapy, friends

You're not failing. Fertility is complex and somewhat random. Give yourself permission to feel whatever you feel, seek help when you need it, and make decisions that protect your wellbeing.

Part Three: Pregnancy Journey

Chapter 10.0: First Trimester Confirmation

Riley stared at the positive pregnancy test for ten minutes. They'd tried six cycles of insemination, spent thousands of dollars, and nearly given up. Now it was real. Two pink lines. A baby. And immediately, the fear: What if something goes wrong? What if this doesn't stick? What if I can't handle this?

The first trimester is weird. You're pregnant but you don't look pregnant. Your body is doing massive things you can't see. You're exhausted but nobody knows why. And if you're LGBTQ+, you're navigating this while deciding who to tell, how to tell them, and how to handle medical systems that often don't quite get your family.

This chapter covers pregnancy confirmation, early prenatal care, first trimester symptoms, managing dysphoria, what to expect at early visits, disclosure decisions, partner involvement, and miscarriage awareness. If you're newly pregnant or trying to get pregnant, this is your roadmap for the first 13 weeks.

10.1 Confirming Pregnancy

Most people know they're pregnant before a doctor confirms it. Home pregnancy tests detect the hormone hCG (human chorionic gonadotropin) in urine about 12-14 days after conception, roughly when your period would be due.

When to test: If you're tracking ovulation and timed insemination attempts, test approximately 14 days after ovulation or insemination. Testing earlier often gives false negatives because hCG levels haven't risen enough to detect yet. If you're using IVF, your clinic will tell you exactly when to test.

Home pregnancy tests: Buy multiple tests. Test with first morning urine (most concentrated). Follow directions exactly. A positive test is almost always accurate—false positives are rare. False negatives happen if you test too early or don't follow directions.

Blood tests: Your provider can order blood tests to measure exact hCG levels. Blood tests detect pregnancy earlier than urine tests and provide quantitative data. Early in pregnancy, hCG should roughly double every 48-72 hours. Providers sometimes order two blood tests a few days apart to confirm levels are rising appropriately.

For LGBTQ+ people specifically: If you've been paying for insemination attempts or IVF, that positive test represents financial investment and emotional energy on top of the usual pregnancy excitement and fear. Let yourself feel whatever you feel—joy, relief, terror, all of it.

If you're a transgender man, that positive test might trigger complex feelings. Relief that it worked, but also dread about what's ahead with dysphoria and being off testosterone longer. Those feelings coexist and both are valid.

10.2 Early Prenatal Care

Once pregnancy is confirmed, schedule your first prenatal visit. Most providers see patients around 8-10 weeks for the first appointment, though this varies.

Choosing providers: If you haven't already chosen your prenatal care provider (covered in Chapter 3.0), do this now. You need someone for the next nine months who respects your identity and understands LGBTQ+ families.

First prenatal visit includes:

- Medical history review (your health, family health history, previous pregnancies)

- Physical exam including blood pressure, weight, sometimes pelvic exam
- Estimated due date calculation (based on last menstrual period or conception date)
- Blood work (blood type, Rh factor, immunity to certain diseases, STI screening, complete blood count, sometimes genetic carrier screening)
- Discussion of what to expect, symptoms, warning signs
- Prescription for prenatal vitamins if you're not already taking them

Early ultrasound: Around 8-10 weeks, you'll likely have an ultrasound to confirm pregnancy location (making sure it's in the uterus and not ectopic), check for heartbeat, and refine due date. Seeing that tiny flickering heartbeat on ultrasound makes pregnancy feel suddenly very real.

For transgender men: First appointments can trigger dysphoria because they involve intimate examination and discussions of anatomy. Remind providers of your pronouns and preferred language before appointments start. Bring your partner or a support person if that helps.

10.3 First Trimester Symptoms

Early pregnancy symptoms vary wildly. Some people feel nothing. Others feel terrible from week six onward. Neither means anything is wrong or right—just different bodies.

Common first trimester symptoms:

Fatigue: Profound, soul-crushing exhaustion is normal. Your body is building a placenta, increasing blood volume, and growing a human. That takes energy. Naps become necessary. Eight hours of sleep isn't enough. You fall asleep on the couch at 7pm. This is all normal (American College of Obstetricians and Gynecologists, 2023).

Nausea and vomiting: About 70-80% of pregnant people experience nausea, and about half vomit (Gadsby et al., 1993). "Morning sickness" is a misnomer—it happens any time. For most people, it peaks around weeks 9-10 and resolves by weeks 12-14. For some unlucky folks, it continues throughout pregnancy.

Strategies that sometimes help: eat small frequent meals, avoid empty stomach, try ginger or peppermint, eat whatever you can tolerate, stay hydrated. If you're vomiting multiple times daily or can't keep fluids down, contact your provider—you might have hyperemesis gravidarum requiring treatment.

Breast/chest tenderness: Hormones cause breast/chest tissue to swell and become tender or painful. For transgender men and non-binary people who've had top surgery, you might not experience this. For those who haven't, it can trigger dysphoria. Wearing a supportive bra or sports bra helps some people.

Frequent urination: Your uterus presses on your bladder, and increased blood flow to the area increases urine production. You'll pee constantly. This is annoying but normal.

Food aversions and cravings: Suddenly you can't stand foods you previously loved, and you desperately want foods you normally ignore. Smell sensitivity increases—things smell overwhelmingly strong. All normal.

Emotional changes: Hormones affect mood. You might cry at commercials, feel irritable, experience anxiety, or have emotional swings. This is expected and usually improves after the first trimester.

Minimal or no symptoms: Some people feel essentially normal throughout the first trimester. This doesn't mean anything is wrong. Lack of symptoms doesn't predict miscarriage risk.

10.4 Managing Dysphoria Early

For transgender men and non-binary pregnant people, first trimester dysphoria can be intense because your body is changing in feminine-coded ways while not yet looking visibly pregnant.

Common dysphoria triggers:

- Breast/chest swelling and tenderness
- Nausea being referred to as "morning sickness" (gendered language)
- Medical providers using feminine language
- Prenatal vitamin bottles with pregnant women on them
- Pregnancy apps with gendered content
- Beginning to show but being misgendered as just gaining weight

Coping strategies:

Reframe mentally: Some transgender men find it helpful to view pregnancy as an intensely masculine experience—using their male body's capacity to create life. Others mentally separate "pregnant body doing pregnancy things" from "my identity as a man." Find what works for you.

Control what you can: Use gender-neutral pregnancy apps (Ovia, for example, allows customization). Ask your provider to use male pronouns and "chest" instead of "breasts" consistently. Remove yourself from gendered pregnancy groups online if they trigger dysphoria.

Therapy support: If you're not already working with a therapist who understands transgender pregnancy, start now. Having professional support for dysphoria management matters.

Community connection: Connect with other transgender men who've been pregnant. Online communities exist specifically for trans pregnancy. You're not alone, even though it feels rare.

Set boundaries: Tell people what language you need and what topics are off-limits. If someone keeps calling you "mama" despite corrections, limit contact with them.

10.5 First Trimester Visits

You'll typically see your provider once in the first trimester, around weeks 8-10, unless complications arise or you have high-risk factors requiring more frequent monitoring.

What happens at first prenatal visit:

- Confirmation of pregnancy and due date
- Complete medical history
- Physical exam
- Blood work
- Discussion of symptoms and what's normal
- Guidance on nutrition, exercise, medications to avoid
- Information about prenatal testing options
- Answering your questions

What to ask at first visit:

- What symptoms should worry me? When should I call?
- What medications/supplements are safe?
- How much weight gain is expected?
- What activities should I avoid?
- When is the next appointment?
- Can my partner attend all appointments?

For LGBTQ+ families specifically:

Ask about documentation: "How do you document my partner in your system? Will they receive medical information? Can they attend all appointments?"

Clarify language: "I prefer male pronouns and the term 'chest' rather than 'breasts.' Can you make sure everyone on your team knows this?"

Address potential issues: "If I need to go to the hospital for complications, how do we ensure staff use correct names and pronouns?"

10.6 Disclosure and Coming Out

Deciding who to tell about your pregnancy and when involves unique considerations for LGBTQ+ people.

Typical disclosure timeline:

Weeks 0-6: Usually only you and your partner (if applicable) know. Many people wait to tell anyone until after week 6-8 when risk of early miscarriage decreases.

Weeks 6-12: Some people tell close family and friends, while others wait until after the first trimester. Traditional advice is to wait until week 12 when miscarriage risk drops significantly, but many LGBTQ+ people tell supportive chosen family earlier because they need support through the difficult first trimester.

Week 12+: Common time to make public announcements after first trimester ends and risk decreases.

LGBTQ+ disclosure considerations:

Who gets to know: Not everyone who knows about your pregnancy needs to know your conception method, donor information, or other private details. You control what information you share.

Coming out as pregnant while LGBTQ+: Announcing pregnancy might be the first time some people learn about your sexual orientation or gender identity. For transgender men, pregnancy might out you as trans if people didn't know. Consider whether you're ready for those conversations.

Work disclosure: You're not legally required to tell your employer you're pregnant until you need accommodations or leave, though many people disclose earlier. For LGBTQ+ people in unsupportive work environments, delayed disclosure might protect you from discrimination.

Scripts for disclosure:

For lesbian couples: "We're pregnant! We used a donor and [Name] is carrying. We're due in [month]."

For transgender man: "I wanted to let you know I'm pregnant. I know that might be surprising, but yes, transgender men can become pregnant. I'm due in [month] and will need some time off around then. I'm happy to answer questions if you have them."

For polyamorous families: "We're expecting a baby! [Names] are the parents. The baby is due in [month]."

Handling reactions: Not everyone will react well. Some people will say ignorant things. Some will ask invasive questions. You don't owe anyone detailed explanations. Prepared responses help:

"Yes, transgender men can become pregnant." "We're not sharing details about conception—that's private." "All three of us are parents to this child." "I use male pronouns, even though I'm pregnant."

10.7 Partner Involvement

Non-gestational partners often feel left out during the first trimester because physical symptoms happen to the pregnant person, not them.

Ways partners can be involved:

Attend appointments: Go to every prenatal appointment you're allowed to attend (some quick check-ins might be gestational-parent-only, but most appointments welcome partners). Being present for ultrasounds, heartbeat checks, and medical discussions helps you feel connected.

Practical support: Make meals when your partner is nauseous, handle chores they're too exhausted to do, grocery shop for whatever foods they can tolerate, take over tasks that trigger their sensitive smell.

Emotional support: Check in about fears and feelings, validate difficult symptoms without trying to fix them, celebrate milestones together (first appointment, first ultrasound, making it to week 12).

Learn together: Read pregnancy books together, follow along with week-by-week fetal development, discuss what's ahead.

For lesbian couples specifically: The non-gestational mother is equally a parent from conception. Make sure medical providers, family, and friends treat both of you as parents, not one parent and one support person. This matters enormously for long-term family dynamics (Goldberg & Perry-Jenkins, 2007).

For transgender men with partners: Your partner needs to advocate for you with medical providers around pronouns and names. Having them do the correcting reduces your emotional labor.

10.8 Miscarriage Awareness

Miscarriage is common in the first trimester. About 10-20% of known pregnancies end in miscarriage, with most occurring before week 12 (American College of Obstetricians and Gynecologists, 2023). After seeing a heartbeat around week 8-10, risk drops significantly to about 5%.

Warning signs of miscarriage:

- Heavy bleeding (soaking through a pad in an hour)
- Severe cramping
- Passing tissue or clots
- Sudden loss of all pregnancy symptoms

Light spotting is common in early pregnancy and doesn't necessarily mean miscarriage. But heavy bleeding or severe pain warrants immediate medical attention.

If miscarriage occurs: It's devastating. Even wanted pregnancies that end early cause profound grief. For LGBTQ+ families who've spent thousands of dollars and significant emotional energy on conception, miscarriage feels especially cruel.

You're allowed to grieve however you need to grieve. You're allowed to be angry about the money lost. You're allowed to feel anything you feel.

Medical management involves either waiting for the pregnancy to pass naturally, taking medication to speed the process, or surgical intervention (D&C) to remove tissue. All three options work and have different benefits and risks.

After miscarriage, most people can try again after one menstrual cycle. But you need time to heal emotionally too. Don't rush into trying again if you're not ready.

Support after miscarriage: Connect with miscarriage support groups, including LGBTQ+ specific groups if available. Consider therapy. Let yourself grieve. Tell people who knew about the pregnancy so they don't keep asking how it's going. Give yourself permission to feel however you feel about trying again.

10.9 Moving Through First Trimester

Consider this composite example: Alex, a non-binary person, confirmed their pregnancy at week six. They told their wife Riley immediately and their closest friends by week seven because they needed support through terrible nausea. They chose a midwife who uses they/them pronouns correctly and refers to Alex's body neutrally.

Alex's first trimester involved exhaustion so profound they napped twice daily, nausea that made everything except saltines and ginger ale intolerable, and dysphoria triggered by chest soreness and being too sick to bind. Riley took over cooking, reminded Alex that this was temporary, and corrected anyone who used wrong pronouns.

At the 10-week appointment, they saw their baby on ultrasound—tiny, moving, with a flickering heartbeat. Alex cried, both from joy and from fear that something would go wrong. The midwife reassured them that everything looked perfect.

They decided to wait until week 13 to tell extended family and make public announcements. By week 12, nausea was improving. By week 13, energy was returning. And they started feeling hopeful that this pregnancy would continue.

10.10 Essential First Trimester Points

The first trimester is physically and emotionally intense. Fatigue, nausea, emotional swings, and body changes are normal. Most symptoms improve significantly after week 12-13. Early prenatal care establishes your relationship with your provider and confirms pregnancy health.

For LGBTQ+ families, first trimester involves decisions about disclosure, managing provider relationships around pronouns and family structure, and supporting non-gestational partners in staying involved. For transgender and non-binary people, early dysphoria management and therapy support matter.

Miscarriage is common in the first trimester. If it happens, grief is legitimate and support is necessary. Most people who experience first trimester miscarriage go on to have successful subsequent pregnancies.

The first trimester is hard. It gets better in the second trimester (Chapter 11.0).

Chapter 11.0: Second Trimester Growth

The nausea lifted around week 14. Elena could finally eat real food again. Energy returned. She felt human for the first time in months. And then, at week 18, she felt it—a flutter. Tiny, unmistakable movement. The baby. Her baby. Their baby. She grabbed Jasmine's hand and held it to her belly, even though it was too early for Jasmine to feel anything from the outside. "The baby just moved," Elena whispered. They both cried.

The second trimester is often called the "honeymoon phase" of pregnancy. For many people, symptoms improve dramatically, energy returns, and you start looking visibly pregnant rather than just tired and bloated. You feel fetal movement. You have the anatomy scan where you might learn baby's sex. You tell everyone, announcing your growing family to the world.

This chapter covers second trimester physical changes, prenatal testing decisions, the anatomy scan, feeling movement, managing dysphoria as your body changes, partner bonding, working while pregnant as an LGBTQ+ person, and making public announcements about your pregnancy.

11.1 Physical Changes

The second trimester (weeks 14-27) brings visible changes as your body grows to accommodate a rapidly developing fetus.

Your growing belly: By week 16-20, most people show visibly. By week 24-27, there's no hiding it—you're obviously pregnant. Your uterus expands from pelvic cavity into abdominal cavity, creating that distinctive pregnant belly.

Weight gain: Expected weight gain is about 1-2 pounds per week in the second and third trimesters (Institute of Medicine, 2009). Total second trimester weight gain is typically 10-15 pounds, though this varies based on pre-pregnancy weight and individual factors.

Some people gain weight easily. Others struggle to gain enough. As long as your provider says growth is appropriate and the baby is measuring well, try not to obsess over the specific numbers.

Skin changes: A dark line (linea nigra) might appear down the center of your belly. Darker patches might appear on your face (melasma or "pregnancy mask"). These are hormonal and usually fade postpartum. Stretch marks often develop as skin stretches over your growing belly—genetics determine susceptibility more than lotions do.

Breast/chest changes: Breast or chest tissue continues growing, preparing for potential feeding. You might leak colostrum (early milk) during the second trimester. For transgender men who haven't had top surgery, this can be distressing.

Movement and balance: As your center of gravity shifts forward, balance changes. You might feel clumsy or trip more easily. This is normal and intensifies in the third trimester.

Energy returns: Most people feel significantly better in the second trimester compared to the first. Nausea resolves. Energy returns. You can function like a human again rather than a exhausted, nauseated zombie.

11.2 Prenatal Testing Decisions

The second trimester involves several prenatal tests that screen for genetic conditions, anatomical abnormalities, and other concerns. You get to decide what testing you want.

Quad screen or integrated screen (15-20 weeks): Blood tests that assess risk of chromosomal abnormalities (Down syndrome, trisomy

18) and neural tube defects. These are screening tests, not diagnostic tests—they give probabilities, not definitive answers. Abnormal screens require follow-up with diagnostic testing.

Anatomy scan (18-22 weeks): Detailed ultrasound examining fetal anatomy—brain, heart, spine, kidneys, limbs, and other structures. This scan checks for major structural abnormalities. It also reveals placenta location and can identify fetal sex if you want to know.

Cell-free DNA testing (available from week 10 onward, but often done second trimester): Non-invasive blood test that analyzes fetal DNA from mother's blood. More accurate than quad screen for chromosomal abnormalities. Can reveal fetal sex. Not all insurance covers it.

Amniocentesis (15-20 weeks): Diagnostic test where fluid is removed from amniotic sac and tested for chromosomal abnormalities and genetic conditions. Carries small risk of miscarriage (about 1 in 300-500). Usually offered if screening tests are abnormal or if you're at increased risk.

Decision-making framework:

Ask yourself: What would we do with the information? If you would terminate pregnancy for certain conditions, testing makes sense. If you wouldn't terminate but would prepare differently or make different birth plans, testing still provides useful information. If you wouldn't change anything based on results, you might skip optional screening.

Consider your risk factors: Age, family history, ethnicity, and previous pregnancy history affect risk of genetic conditions. Your provider can explain your specific risk profile.

For LGBTQ+ families: These decisions belong to whoever will be legal parents. If you're co-parenting or in a polyamorous arrangement, make sure everyone with parental rights participates in decisions about testing.

11.3 The Anatomy Scan

Around weeks 18-22, you'll have a detailed anatomy ultrasound. This is often the most exciting appointment of pregnancy because you see your baby in detail, moving around, sucking their thumb, doing flips.

What the scan examines:

- Brain structure and development
- Face and profile
- Spine alignment
- Four-chamber heart view
- Stomach, kidneys, bladder
- Arms, legs, fingers, toes
- Placenta location
- Amniotic fluid levels
- Fetal measurements and growth

The sonographer looks for structural abnormalities. Most scans show normal development. Occasionally, concerns arise requiring follow-up with specialists.

Learning baby's sex: The anatomy scan can identify fetal sex if you want to know. Some families want to know. Others prefer surprises. Both are fine.

For LGBTQ+ families, finding out sex might feel more complicated. Some families worry about gender expectations or imposing binary gender on a child before they can express their own identity. Others want to know for practical planning. There's no right answer—just what feels right for your family.

Gender reveal considerations: If you do learn the sex and want to tell people, consider whether you want a gender reveal party. Some LGBTQ+ families skip them entirely because they reinforce gender binaries. Others have them but explicitly frame them as "sex reveal" parties (biological sex at birth, not gender). Others fully embrace the tradition. Do what feels authentic to you.

11.4 Feeling Movement

Somewhere between weeks 16-25 (most commonly 18-20 for first pregnancies, earlier for subsequent pregnancies), you'll feel your baby move for the first time. It's called "quickening" and it's magical.

What early movement feels like: Flutters, bubbles, gentle tapping. It's subtle. Many people initially mistake it for gas or digestive movements. But once you know what it is, you'll recognize it instantly.

Movement increases: As pregnancy progresses, movements become stronger, more frequent, and more obvious. By the third trimester, you'll feel distinct kicks, punches, rolls, and stretches. Non-pregnant people can feel baby move by placing hands on your belly.

Bonding through movement: Feeling your baby move creates tangible connection. This is a real person growing inside you. For many pregnant people, movement makes pregnancy feel real in a way ultrasounds don't.

For non-gestational partners: Eventually, you'll be able to feel baby move from the outside by placing your hand on your partner's belly. This often starts around weeks 24-28 depending on baby's position and activity. It's one of the few ways non-gestational parents can physically interact with the baby before birth.

11.5 Dysphoria and Body Changes

For transgender men and non-binary people, the second trimester often brings increased dysphoria because your body becomes visibly, undeniably pregnant.

Dysphoria triggers in second trimester:

- Visible pregnant belly
- Strangers gendering you as female based on pregnancy
- Maternity clothes (designed for women)
- People touching your belly without asking
- Comments like "You're glowing!" or other feminine-coded pregnancy language
- Breast/chest growth
- Feeling trapped in a body that looks increasingly feminine

Strategies for managing:

Clothing choices: Wear clothes that feel authentic to you. Oversized hoodies, men's t-shirts stretched over belly, maternity pants with masculine tops. You don't have to wear feminine maternity clothes.

Boundary setting: Tell people not to touch your belly. Practice saying: "Please don't touch me without asking." Most people respect boundaries when you set them clearly.

Reframe mentally: Some transgender men find it helpful to view their pregnant body as their male body doing something male bodies with uteruses can do. It's not a female experience—it's your masculine experience of pregnancy. Others mentally separate body and identity. Find the framework that works for you.

Limit exposure: If seeing pregnant women triggers dysphoria (by comparison or by highlighting how others perceive you), limit time in spaces full of visibly pregnant people.

Therapy and community: Continue therapy. Stay connected to other transgender people who've been pregnant. You're not alone in this difficult experience.

11.6 Partner Bonding

Non-gestational partners often feel more connected in the second trimester because pregnancy becomes visible and baby's movements become feelable.

Ways non-gestational partners bond with baby:

Attend anatomy scan: Seeing your baby in detail on ultrasound makes them real. Watching them move, seeing their face (sort of—ultrasound images are grainy), noting their measurements—this creates connection.

Feel movement: Once movement is strong enough to feel from outside, spend time with your hand on your partner's belly. Talk to the baby. They can hear you from about 18-20 weeks onward.

Prepare together: Start planning nursery, buying baby items, making decisions about gear and childcare and feeding. These activities involve both partners equally.

Read pregnancy books together: Follow fetal development week by week. Learn what's happening inside your partner's body. Understand what they're experiencing physically.

Take classes together: Many areas offer prenatal classes (childbirth education, infant care, feeding classes). Attending together prepares you both for what's ahead.

Talk about parenting: Discuss your values, your hopes, your fears about parenthood. Align on approaches to discipline, education, religion, how you'll divide childcare labor, and how you'll handle disagreements.

11.7 Working While Pregnant

Being visibly pregnant at work brings unique challenges for LGBTQ+ people because pregnancy might out you or create awkward conversations.

For lesbian and queer women: You might field questions about baby's father or assumptions about your relationship status. Responses: "We used a donor." "My wife and I are both the mothers." You don't owe lengthy explanations.

For transgender men: Pregnancy visibility might out you as trans to colleagues who didn't know. This can trigger dysphoria and create safety concerns depending on your workplace. You might need to have conversations you weren't planning to have.

For non-binary people: Visible pregnancy often causes people to gender you female regardless of your actual identity or presentation. Constantly being misgendered at work is exhausting.

Legal protections: Pregnancy discrimination is illegal under federal law (Pregnancy Discrimination Act). You cannot be fired, demoted, or denied opportunities because of pregnancy. You're entitled to the same accommodations provided to other temporarily disabled workers—modified duties, breaks, flexible schedule if needed (U.S. Equal Employment Opportunity Commission, 2023).

LGBTQ+ discrimination is increasingly protected (post-Bostock v. Clayton County), but enforcement varies by location. Document any discrimination you experience.

Telling your employer: When you tell your employer you're pregnant depends on your circumstances. Many people wait until after the first trimester but before it's obvious. You're not legally required to disclose until you need accommodations or request leave.

Plan what you'll say: "I wanted to let you know I'm pregnant. I'm due in [month]. I'll need [length] of leave around my due date. I'm happy to discuss transition plans."

Dealing with invasive questions: Coworkers often ask inappropriate questions. You can deflect: "That's pretty personal," or give minimal information: "We're excited about the baby." You don't owe details about conception, donor information, or your sexual orientation or gender identity.

11.8 Public Announcements

Most people make public pregnancy announcements after the first trimester, typically between weeks 12-20. Social media announcements, telling extended family, informing broader social circles—this is when pregnancy becomes public knowledge.

Announcement considerations for LGBTQ+ families:

How much to share: You control the narrative. Announce your pregnancy however feels right: "We're pregnant!" "We're expecting a baby in [month]!" "Our family is growing!" You don't have to explain conception methods, donor details, or anything else unless you want to.

Photos: Many pregnancy announcements include photos. Some LGBTQ+ families include both partners in photos to emphasize that you're both parents. Others show just the pregnant person. Some skip photos entirely.

For lesbian couples: Consider whether your announcement makes clear that you're both mothers. "We're expecting our first child" or "We're pregnant with our baby" signals joint parenthood better than "I'm pregnant."

For transgender men: Announcing pregnancy as a visibly male person is a gender-affirming statement. It normalizes transgender pregnancy and might educate people who didn't know trans men could get pregnant. But it also potentially exposes you to harassment or invasive questions. Consider your safety and comfort level.

Social media caution: Once you announce on social media, expect comments. Some will be lovely. Some might be ignorant or hurtful. You can moderate comments, block people, or limit who sees the announcement. Protect your mental health.

11.9 Real World Example

Consider Priya and Nicole's second trimester (composite): They announced their pregnancy at week 13 with a social media post showing both of them holding a onesie that said "Made with love (and science)." They got overwhelmingly positive responses with a few awkward questions about "who's the father."

At their anatomy scan at week 20, they learned they were having a girl. They decided not to do a gender reveal party because it felt too focused on gender stereotypes. Instead, they just told people directly.

Priya started showing obviously by week 18. At work, colleagues congratulated her and asked typical questions. When people said "Dad must be excited," Priya corrected them: "Her other mom is very excited, yes." Most people adjusted quickly.

Nicole felt the baby move from the outside for the first time at week 25. Priya called her over during dinner and placed her hand on her belly. Nicole felt a strong kick and started crying. This was their baby, kicking her hand. She was a mother already, even though the baby wasn't born yet.

By the end of the second trimester, they'd told everyone, bought baby gear, and started preparing the nursery. Priya's energy was good. They were both excited and terrified. The third trimester awaited.

11.10 Key Second Trimester Insights

The second trimester is often the easiest physically, with returned energy and resolved nausea. Your belly grows visibly, you feel fetal movement, and the anatomy scan provides detailed look at your developing baby. Prenatal testing offers information about genetic conditions and abnormalities—you decide what testing feels right for your family.

For LGBTQ+ families, the second trimester involves increased visibility (your pregnancy is obvious), which creates both celebration and challenges. Transgender and non-binary people manage increased dysphoria as body changes intensify. Non-gestational partners bond more readily once they can see and feel baby from the outside. Work situations require navigating disclosure and potential discrimination.

Public announcements make pregnancy official to your broader world. You control how much you share and how you frame your family story. Most people experience the second trimester as hopeful and exciting—the hard first trimester is past, and the uncomfortable third trimester isn't here yet.

Chapter 12.0: Third Trimester Preparation

Marcus hit week 32 and suddenly everything felt urgent. The baby was coming. Soon. They needed to finish the nursery, pack hospital bags, write a birth plan, prepare for labor. But he was also exhausted again, his back hurt constantly, and bending over to tie shoes required strategic planning. The final stretch was hard.

The third trimester (weeks 28-40+) is about preparation—physically preparing your body for labor, practically preparing your home and hospital bag, mentally preparing for birth and parenthood. Your body is finishing growing a human while that human is running out of room, making everything uncomfortable. You're excited and terrified, ready for birth but scared of birth, desperate to meet your baby but not sure if you're actually ready to be a parent.

This chapter covers preparing for labor, nesting and home preparation, birth planning for LGBTQ+ families, hospital bag packing, late pregnancy discomforts, signs of labor, early labor at home, and partner preparation for supporting labor.

12.1 Preparing Your Body

Labor is intense physical work. Your body prepares throughout the third trimester, but you can actively support readiness.

Practice positions: Try various positions that might help during labor—squatting, hands and knees, side-lying, standing and swaying. Practice these weekly so they feel natural.

Pelvic floor exercises: Kegel exercises (tightening and releasing pelvic floor muscles) help you connect with muscles used during pushing. But also practice releasing and relaxing these muscles—birth requires letting go, not clenching.

Perineal massage (starting around week 34): Gentle massage of perineal tissue (the area between vagina and anus) with oil or lubricant can increase tissue flexibility and potentially reduce tearing during birth. Research shows modest benefit (Beckmann & Stock, 2013). Some people do this themselves, others ask partners to help.

Stay active: Walking, swimming, prenatal yoga—movement keeps you strong and helps baby move into good position for birth. But don't push yourself too hard. Listen to your body.

Rest: You also need rest. Lots of rest. Sleep whenever possible because sleep becomes scarce once baby arrives. Nap. Go to bed early. Rest is preparation too.

Nutrition: Eat well. Stay hydrated. Your body needs fuel for labor and for building final reserves before birth. Dates might help—one small study suggested eating dates in late pregnancy might reduce need for induction, though evidence is limited (Al-Kuran et al., 2011).

12.2 Nesting and Home Preparation

"Nesting" is the urge to prepare your home for baby—cleaning, organizing, arranging. It's real and often intensifies in the final weeks.

Baby essentials to have ready:

- Place for baby to sleep (bassinet, crib, co-sleeper)
- Diapers and wipes
- Several changes of clothes in newborn and 0-3 month sizes
- Swaddle blankets
- Feeding supplies (bottles, formula if planning to use it, nursing pillow if chest/breastfeeding)

- Car seat (required to leave hospital—practice installing it before labor)
- Basic bath supplies

Prepare your space:

- Set up changing area
- Arrange nursery if you have one (though baby will likely sleep in your room initially)
- Stock your fridge and pantry with easy meals
- Do laundry and clean house before labor (it's absurdly satisfying)
- Set up stations around the house with baby supplies so you don't have to climb stairs constantly

Prepare for postpartum:

- Stock postpartum supplies (heavy pads, witch hazel pads, pain relief, stool softeners)
- Make and freeze meals
- Line up help for the first weeks
- Prep easy snacks for middle-of-night feeding sessions

For non-gestational partners: You can do most physical preparation since your partner is increasingly uncomfortable. Take over the nesting activities—it helps you feel useful and gives your partner rest.

12.3 Birth Planning

Birth plans (sometimes called birth preferences) communicate your hopes for labor and birth to your care team. They're not binding contracts—labor doesn't always go as planned—but they guide decisions.

Components of inclusive birth plan:

Language preferences: Specify pronouns for the pregnant person, terms for anatomy (chest vs. breasts, pregnant person vs. mother), titles for partners (mother, father, parent).

Pain management preferences: Unmedicated birth, epidural only if requested, open to all options. State your preferences while acknowledging flexibility if circumstances change.

Movement and positions: Preference to move freely during labor, try various positions, labor in water if available.

Partner involvement: Who will be present (partner, doula, other support people), their roles during labor, who cuts the cord.

Interventions: Preferences about monitoring (intermittent vs. continuous), IV vs. saline lock, when you want interventions suggested.

Pushing and birth: Preferences about coached pushing vs. spontaneous pushing, positions for birth, immediate skin-to-skin vs. brief evaluation then skin-to-skin.

Cesarean preferences if necessary: Gentle cesarean techniques, partner present, skin-to-skin in operating room, which partner accompanies baby to nursery.

Immediate postpartum: Delayed cord clamping, who holds baby first, chest/breastfeeding immediately vs. bottle first, rooming in vs. nursery care.

Newborn procedures: Vitamin K injection, eye ointment, hepatitis B vaccine, circumcision if applicable—consent or decline for each.

LGBTQ+ specific considerations: Explicitly state pronouns, partner titles, that you want staff to use inclusive language, that both/all parents should receive equal information and respect, any specific concerns about discrimination or misgendering.

12.4 Hospital Bag Packing

Around week 36, pack bags for the hospital (or birth center). You'll want three bags: one for labor, one for postpartum recovery, one for baby.

Labor bag:

- Comfortable clothes or labor gown
- Snacks (unless your provider prohibits eating in labor)
- Drinks with straws or sports bottles
- Phone and charger
- Music or entertainment
- Chapstick, hair ties, massage oil or lotion
- Birth plan copies (several—give to every shift)
- Comfort items (photos, inspiring quotes, whatever helps)

Postpartum bag:

- Going-home outfit (you'll still look pregnant—bring maternity clothes)
- Toiletries (toothbrush, shampoo, face wash, etc.)
- Comfortable underwear you don't mind ruining or disposable underwear
- Nursing bra or comfortable bra if chest/breastfeeding
- Slippers or comfortable shoes
- Robe for walking halls
- Phone charger
- Entertainment (books, tablet)

Baby bag:

- Going-home outfit (bring two sizes—newborn and 0-3 months—babies vary)
- Blanket for car seat
- Diapers and wipes (hospital provides these but having your own doesn't hurt)
- Car seat (installed in car before labor)

Partner bag:

- Change of clothes
- Toiletries
- Snacks
- Phone charger
- Entertainment for long labor
- Pillow and blanket if sleeping at hospital
- Cash for vending machines and parking

LGBTQ+ specific items:

- Multiple copies of birth plan emphasizing pronouns and family structure
- Names and numbers for patient advocates if discrimination occurs
- Legal documents establishing partner's parental status if available
- Anything that helps you feel comfortable and affirmed

12.5 Late Pregnancy Discomforts

The third trimester is uncomfortable. There's no getting around it. Your body is enormous, the baby is running out of room, and everything hurts.

Common complaints:

Back pain: Your center of gravity shifted forward, straining back muscles. Prenatal massage helps. Warm baths help. Supportive pillows help. But mostly you just endure.

Pelvic pressure and pain: Baby's head pressing into your pelvis causes achiness. Sometimes you feel like baby might fall out (they won't, but it feels that way).

Shortness of breath: Baby is crowding your lungs. You get winded walking across the room. This improves once baby "drops" into the pelvis, usually a few weeks before birth for first pregnancies.

Frequent urination returns: Baby presses on your bladder. You pee constantly, including multiple times per night.

Insomnia: Despite exhaustion, sleeping is hard. You can't get comfortable. You have to pee constantly. Your mind races. Sleep deprivation before labor is cruel but common.

Braxton Hicks contractions: Practice contractions that tighten your belly irregularly. They're uncomfortable but not progressive. If they become regular (every 5-10 minutes for an hour), call your provider.

Swelling: Feet and ankles swell. Hands swell. Your rings might not fit. Elevate feet when possible. Drink water. This is normal unless accompanied by severe headaches or visual changes (signs of preeclampsia requiring immediate medical attention).

Heartburn: Baby pushes your stomach upward. Acid reflux is miserable. Antacids help. Eating small frequent meals helps. Sleeping propped up helps.

12.6 When to Go In

Around week 36, your provider will review signs of labor and when to go to hospital or birth center.

Signs to call provider or go to hospital:

Regular contractions: For first babies, typical guideline is "5-1-1 rule"—contractions every 5 minutes, lasting 1 minute each, for 1 hour. For subsequent babies, often earlier because labor progresses faster.

Water breaking: If your bag of waters breaks (gush or trickle of fluid), call your provider. Many people need to deliver within 24 hours after water breaks to reduce infection risk.

Severe bleeding: Light bloody show is normal in early labor. Heavy bleeding requires immediate evaluation.

Decreased fetal movement: If baby stops moving or movement decreases significantly, go to hospital for monitoring.

Severe pain: Labor contractions are painful but come and go. Constant severe pain might indicate complications.

Signs of preeclampsia: Severe headache, visual changes (spots, blurriness), severe swelling, pain under ribs. These require immediate evaluation.

Your gut feeling: If something feels wrong, go in. Better to be checked and sent home than to ignore warning signs.

12.7 Early Labor at Home

Early labor is typically spent at home. Going to hospital too early often leads to interventions. Stay home as long as safely possible.

Early labor signs:

- Regular contractions that gradually intensify and get closer together
- Possible bloody show (mucus plug tinged with blood)
- Possible water breaking (though water breaks before contractions for only about 10% of people)
- Cramping similar to menstrual cramps
- Backache
- Burst of energy (nesting urge intensifies)
- Loose bowels

Coping during early labor at home:

- Rest if it's night or you're tired—you'll need energy later
- Stay active if you're alert—walk, sway, stay upright
- Eat light foods and stay hydrated
- Time contractions when they become regular (several apps make this easy)
- Distract yourself—watch movies, take a bath, do light activities
- Use comfort measures—heating pad, massage, position changes

When to go to hospital: Follow the guidelines your provider gave you, typically 5-1-1 for first babies or when contractions are intense enough that you can't walk or talk through them.

12.8 Partner Preparation

Partners need preparation for how to support labor. This matters enormously for the laboring person's experience.

What partners should learn:

- Stages of labor and what to expect
- Comfort measures (massage, counterpressure, position suggestions, breathing reminders)
- When to call provider or go to hospital
- Signs of complications
- How to be present emotionally without being overwhelming
- When to advocate and what to advocate for

Take childbirth education class together: Many areas offer classes covering labor stages, comfort measures, medical interventions, postpartum care. These prepare you both.

Read birth books together: Books like *The Birth Partner* by Penny Simkin specifically guide partners through supporting labor.

Practice comfort measures: Try different massage techniques, practice breathing together, discuss what might help during intense contractions.

Make plans: Discuss when to call provider, when to go to hospital, who will watch other children or pets, what to do if labor starts while you're apart.

For non-gestational partners specifically: Labor is your time to actively support. This is when you can finally do something concrete after months of watching your partner be pregnant. Prepare well. Your presence and support matter enormously.

12.9 Final Weeks Example

Consider Jordan and Taylor's preparation (composite): At week 36, Jordan, who is carrying, suddenly became obsessed with cleaning. Taylor came home to find Jordan scrubbing baseboards at 10pm. Nesting was real.

They packed hospital bags, installed the car seat (took an hour and three YouTube videos to get it right), and attended a childbirth class. Taylor practiced counterpressure on Jordan's lower back because Jordan's back labor in previous pregnancy had been terrible.

Jordan's birth plan specified they/them pronouns, gender-neutral language, and that Taylor was equally a parent entitled to all information. They made copies for every medical shift.

At week 38, Jordan's Braxton Hicks contractions became intense. They went to hospital thinking labor had started. They were sent home—false alarm. Embarrassing but common.

Real labor started at week 39+3. Contractions woke Jordan at 3am. They labored at home until 7am when contractions were five minutes apart and impossible to talk through. Taylor drove them to hospital. Their baby was born 12 hours later.

12.10 Preparation Essentials

The third trimester is physically uncomfortable but practically productive. Prepare your body through gentle exercise, positioning practice, and rest. Prepare your home through nesting activities and gathering supplies. Create a birth plan that communicates your preferences and LGBTQ+ specific needs. Pack hospital bags. Learn signs of labor and when to go in.

Early labor is typically spent at home using comfort measures and staying nourished and hydrated. Partners prepare by learning comfort techniques and labor support strategies. Everyone prepares mentally for the intensity ahead.

Late pregnancy is the final countdown. You're ready to meet your baby. You're terrified of labor. You're excited about parenthood. You're exhausted from being pregnant. All of this coexists as you approach birth.

Chapter 13.0: Trans Pregnancy Care

Kai's first prenatal appointment as a pregnant transgender man went better than expected. The midwife used his pronouns correctly, referred to his chest rather than breasts, and never once seemed surprised or confused that a man was pregnant. But at the ultrasound, the technician kept saying "mom" despite corrections. Then the lab tech called him "miss." By the time he left, he was exhausted from constant corrections and felt more dysphoric than he had in years.

Transgender and non-binary pregnant people face unique challenges in prenatal care: navigating gendered medical systems, managing dysphoria throughout pregnancy, finding truly competent providers, and advocating for correct pronouns and language when you're physically vulnerable. This chapter provides specific guidance for trans and non-binary pregnancy experiences, covering provider selection, managing pelvic exams, chest changes, documentation issues, advocacy strategies, mental health support, and testosterone monitoring.

13.1 Finding Trans Competent Providers

Not all providers who say they're LGBTQ+-affirming actually understand transgender pregnancy. You need providers who have specific experience with trans pregnancy and won't treat you like an educational burden.

What trans competency looks like:

- Immediate correct pronoun use after you state them once
- Natural use of your preferred anatomy terms without discomfort

- Knowledge about testosterone's effects on pregnancy
- Understanding of dysphoria and how to minimize triggers
- Experience with other trans pregnant patients
- Advocacy for you with other staff
- Zero surprise or discomfort about your male/non-binary identity while pregnant

Questions to ask potential providers:

- How many transgender or non-binary pregnant people have you cared for?
- What training have you received in trans perinatal health?
- How do you handle documentation when gender markers don't match reproductive anatomy?
- What's your approach to using gender-neutral or masculine language during pregnancy care?
- How do you prepare hospital staff for transgender patients during labor?
- Can you provide references from other trans clients?

Red flags:

- Repeated pronoun mistakes
- Visible discomfort with your identity
- Lack of knowledge about testosterone and pregnancy
- Treating your pregnancy as unusual or shocking
- Requiring you to educate them about basic trans concepts
- Resistance to using your preferred language

Where to find trans-competent providers: Ask other transgender men or non-binary people who've been pregnant for recommendations. Check the World Professional Association for Transgender Health provider directory. Look for practices that specifically advertise trans pregnancy care. Urban areas in progressive states generally have more options, though telehealth expands access (WPATH, 2023).

13.2 Gendered vs Neutral Providers

Some transgender pregnant people prefer providers who use exclusively gender-neutral language. Others are comfortable with some gendered language as long as it's applied correctly (calling you "father" not "mother," for instance). Neither preference is more valid.

Gender-neutral approach: Provider uses terms like "pregnant person," "birthing person," "chest," "lower anatomy," "gestational parent." All materials and language avoid gender entirely.

Correctly gendered approach: Provider uses masculine language for you specifically while maintaining medical accuracy—"You're a man having a baby," "Your chest might be sore," "You'll be a father soon."

What matters: Your provider uses the language you specify. If you want neutral language, they should use neutral language. If you want masculine language, they should use masculine language. This is about your comfort, not their assumptions.

13.3 Pelvic Exams and Dysphoria

Pelvic exams are standard during pregnancy: checking cervix, monitoring fetal position, assessing dilation late in pregnancy. For many transgender men and non-binary people, pelvic exams trigger intense dysphoria.

Strategies for managing dysphoria during exams:

Communicate needs upfront: Before the exam, tell your provider: "Pelvic exams trigger dysphoria for me. Can we minimize these to only what's medically necessary? When they're necessary, can you talk me through what you're doing and check in with me?"

Use correct language: Ask your provider to use your preferred terms for anatomy. If "vagina" triggers dysphoria, use "front hole" or "lower anatomy" or whatever term feels neutral or affirming to you.

Bring support: Have your partner present during exams if that helps. They can hold your hand, remind you to breathe, and provide distraction.

Distraction techniques: Bring headphones and music, focus on breathing, count ceiling tiles, ask your provider to talk about something unrelated while examining you.

Minimize exams: Not every prenatal visit requires a pelvic exam. Ask what's medically necessary versus routine. Skip routine exams if they're not essential.

Take breaks: If dysphoria becomes overwhelming during an exam, say "Stop. I need a minute." Good providers will pause, check in, and proceed only when you're ready.

Consider this perspective from research: Transgender men report that being treated as men during pregnancy—having their identity respected and affirmed—reduces trauma and improves care experiences even when procedures themselves trigger dysphoria (Hoffkling et al., 2017).

13.4 Chest Changes

Pregnancy causes breast/chest tissue to swell, become tender, and prepare for potential lactation. For transgender men, especially those who haven't had top surgery, chest changes can be distressing.

What to expect:

- Swelling and tenderness throughout pregnancy
- Darkening of areolas
- Possible leaking of colostrum in second and third trimesters
- Significant size increase
- Continued changes postpartum if chest-feeding

Managing chest dysphoria:

Clothing: Wear loose clothing or compression garments if comfortable (though not tight binding during pregnancy as this can restrict breathing and blood flow).

Avoid mirrors: If seeing your chest triggers dysphoria, minimize exposure. Shower with eyes closed or averted, dress quickly, avoid full-length mirrors.

Reframe mentally: Some transgender men find it helpful to think of chest changes as functional rather than gendered—"My chest is producing food for my baby" rather than "I'm developing breasts like a woman."

Plan for after: Knowing you can resume binding or pursue top surgery postpartum (after weaning if you chest-feed) provides endpoint. This is temporary.

Top surgery and pregnancy: If you've had top surgery before pregnancy, you likely won't experience significant chest changes. You won't be able to chest-feed (no mammary tissue remaining), but pregnancy itself won't significantly affect your chest.

13.5 Documentation Issues

Medical systems struggle with documentation when gender markers don't match reproductive anatomy. This creates insurance denials, billing problems, and constant explanations.

Common documentation problems:

- Insurance denying pregnancy-related claims for people with male gender markers
- Medical records systems requiring female gender for OB care
- Birth certificates defaulting to "mother" regardless of your gender
- ID not matching medical records, creating confusion at appointments

Strategies for managing:

Insurance appeals: If insurance denies pregnancy coverage due to gender markers, appeal immediately. Your provider should write letters of medical necessity explaining that transgender men can become pregnant and require pregnancy care. Lambda Legal and the National Center for Transgender Equality provide resources for fighting discriminatory denials (NCTE, 2021).

Multiple names in system: Some medical systems allow both legal name and chosen name. Use this feature so staff see the name you actually use.

Advocate preemptively: Before appointments, call and confirm your name and pronouns are in the system. "I have an appointment tomorrow. My name is Marcus and I use he/him pronouns. Can you make sure that's in my chart?"

Document everything: Keep copies of insurance denials, appeal letters, and communications. You might need evidence of discrimination for legal action or to support policy change.

Birth certificate considerations: Work with attorneys before birth to understand your state's process for getting correct parental designation on birth certificates. Some states allow "father" or "parent" instead of "mother" for transgender men who give birth. Others require court orders to change birth certificates after the fact.

13.6 Advocating for Pronouns

You'll interact with dozens of medical staff during pregnancy—receptionists, nurses, midwives, physicians, ultrasound techs, lab staff. Not everyone will get your pronouns right, even with notes in your chart.

Setting expectations at first contact: When scheduling your first appointment, state clearly: "I'm a transgender man. I use he/him pronouns. Please make sure this is prominently noted in my chart."

This sets precedent that your gender identity is important information.

Correcting mistakes:

Immediate correction: When someone uses wrong pronouns, correct immediately and matter-of-factly: "He, not she." Most people will apologize and correct. Don't make it a big deal unless they repeatedly fail to adjust.

Strategic correction: You don't have to correct every mistake. If you'll never see this person again and correcting will create an awkward situation, sometimes it's easier to let it go. Save your energy for people you'll interact with repeatedly.

Partner advocacy: Have your partner do correcting when possible. "He, actually—my partner uses he/him pronouns." This reduces your emotional labor and signals to staff that respecting pronouns matters to everyone present.

Escalating persistent problems: If the same person repeatedly uses wrong pronouns after multiple corrections, escalate. Talk to their supervisor, notify patient advocates, file formal complaints. Persistent misgendering is discrimination.

13.7 Mental Health Support

Pregnancy as a transgender man or non-binary person is mentally difficult. The physical dysphoria combines with discrimination, lack of community, and the weirdness of doing something typically coded as intensely feminine while being male or non-binary.

Common mental health challenges:

- Intense dysphoria throughout pregnancy
- Isolation (few transgender men get pregnant; you might not know anyone else who's done this)
- Discrimination and microaggressions in healthcare

- Fear about parenting as trans person
- Concerns about how pregnancy will affect transition or identity
- Grief about stopping testosterone
- Anxiety about labor and postpartum

Getting support:

Therapy: Work with a therapist who understands both transgender identity and perinatal issues. Ideally, find someone with experience in transgender pregnancy specifically. If nobody local has this expertise, consider telehealth.

Transgender pregnancy communities: Online groups exist specifically for transgender men and non-binary people who are pregnant or have been pregnant. Reddit communities, Facebook groups, and forums provide peer support and practical advice from people who've been through it.

General pregnancy support (with caution): Regular pregnancy groups can provide practical information but might trigger dysphoria due to gendered language and assumptions. Use them for practical questions, skip the gendered discussion threads.

Partner or family support: Rely on people who affirm your identity and understand your experience. If biological family isn't supportive, chosen family and partner support matter even more.

Medication if needed: Some people need medication for depression or anxiety during pregnancy. Many psychiatric medications are safe in pregnancy. Don't suffer unnecessarily—work with a psychiatrist familiar with pregnancy to find safe options.

13.8 Testosterone Monitoring

If you stopped testosterone to become pregnant, monitoring your health during this time matters.

What happens without testosterone:

- Menstruation returns (stops once pregnant)
- Some masculinizing effects of testosterone persist (voice, facial hair, body hair)
- Some effects may partially reverse (fat redistribution toward hips, slight breast tissue development)
- Mental and emotional effects vary—some people feel fine off testosterone, others struggle with mood changes

Monitoring health: Your prenatal care provider should monitor your overall health. If you experience concerning mood changes or physical symptoms, mention them. Being off testosterone shouldn't cause major health problems, but individual experiences vary.

Resuming testosterone postpartum: You can restart testosterone after pregnancy. If you're chest-feeding, you'll need to wait until weaning (testosterone suppresses milk production and passes through milk). If you're not chest-feeding, you can resume immediately postpartum. Discuss timing with your hormone prescriber.

13.9 Community and Connection

Transgender pregnancy can feel isolating. Finding community matters.

Online spaces: Several active communities exist for trans pregnancy:

- Reddit's r/seahorse_dads (for trans men who are pregnant or have given birth)
- Facebook groups for trans pregnancy
- Instagram accounts documenting trans pregnancy journeys
- Forums on trans health websites

Local connections: LGBTQ+ parenting groups sometimes include transgender parents. Transgender community organizations might connect you with others who've been through pregnancy.

Creating visibility: Some transgender men choose to be public about their pregnancy experiences—posting on social media, writing about it, participating in research or media. This creates visibility and helps normalize trans pregnancy. Others keep pregnancy private. Both approaches are valid. Do what feels safe and authentic for you.

13.10 Real Experience Integration

Consider this composite narrative: Ravi, a 29-year-old transgender man, had been on testosterone for seven years when he decided to pursue pregnancy. Stopping testosterone triggered immediate dysphoria—his period returned after three months, and he felt emotionally fragile in ways he hadn't since before transition.

His midwife practice had never worked with a pregnant trans man before, but they were eager to learn. They consistently used correct pronouns, called him "father," and referred to his "chest" without hesitation. At the hospital, he had to educate everyone repeatedly, but the midwives advocated fiercely for him.

Pregnancy itself was harder than Ravi expected. The chest development triggered severe dysphoria. Being visibly pregnant while male meant constant stares and questions. He stopped going to his gym because the pregnant-man thing made people uncomfortable.

But his partner's unwavering support helped. They attended every appointment, corrected pronouns relentlessly, and reminded Ravi that he was a man doing something only some men's bodies can do—a profoundly masculine act of creating life.

Ravi gave birth at 39 weeks. Labor was intense and triggering—the exposure, the intimate examinations, the physical intensity. But he did it. He became a father. Three months postpartum, after deciding not to chest-feed, he resumed testosterone. Six months postpartum, he barely remembered what dysphoria felt like during pregnancy. His son was worth every difficult moment.

13.11 Key Principles

Transgender and non-binary pregnant people need trans-competent providers who use correct language, understand dysphoria, and advocate with other staff. Pelvic exams trigger dysphoria but can be managed through communication, support, and minimizing unnecessary procedures. Chest changes during pregnancy are distressing for many trans people, requiring mental reframing and planning for postpartum.

Documentation systems create barriers through mismatched gender markers and insurance denials—persistent advocacy and appeals overcome these obstacles. Pronoun misgendering happens frequently; immediate correction and partner advocacy help. Mental health support through therapy and trans pregnancy communities reduces isolation and manages dysphoria throughout pregnancy.

Pregnancy as a transgender or non-binary person is difficult and isolating but possible. Many trans men and non-binary people successfully navigate pregnancy with good support, competent providers, and strong advocacy. You're not alone, even when it feels that way.

Chapter 14.0: Partner Involvement During Pregnancy

Jasmine felt invisible. Elena was pregnant with their baby—their baby—but everyone directed questions to Elena, handed paperwork to Elena, asked how "mom" was feeling while ignoring Jasmine entirely. At the ultrasound, the technician kept calling Elena "mom" and referring to Jasmine as "your friend" despite their wedding rings and repeated corrections. Jasmine left appointments feeling like a spectator in her own family's creation.

Non-gestational partners in LGBTQ+ families face unique challenges: being erased by medical systems, managing feelings of disconnection from pregnancy, navigating external perceptions of your role, and figuring out how to bond with a baby you can't feel moving inside your body. This chapter addresses partner involvement throughout pregnancy, covering bonding strategies, attending appointments, managing external perceptions, co-parenting decisions, supporting the pregnant partner, handling difficult emotions, and preparing siblings.

14.1 Non-Gestational Partner Bonding

When your partner is pregnant but you're not, bonding with the baby requires intention because you don't have the physical connection the pregnant person has.

Strategies for bonding:

Attend all appointments: Be present for every prenatal visit you're allowed to attend. Hearing the heartbeat, seeing ultrasounds, learning about fetal development—these create connection. Request that providers direct information to both of you equally.

Talk to the baby: Once the baby can hear (around 18-20 weeks), talk to them regularly. Read books, sing songs, tell stories. Your voice will be familiar when they're born.

Feel movement: In the second and third trimesters, place your hand on your partner's belly to feel kicks and movements. This tangible interaction helps you connect.

Participate in preparation: Shop for baby items together, set up the nursery, attend childbirth classes, pack hospital bags. These practical activities involve you directly in preparation.

Learn week by week: Follow fetal development in pregnancy apps or books. Know what's happening each week—when fingers develop, when the baby can hear, when they start practicing breathing movements. This helps you feel connected to the growing baby even though you can't feel physical changes.

Create rituals: Some couples create weekly rituals—belly photos, letters to the baby, special dinners—that involve both partners in marking pregnancy milestones.

Research shows: Non-gestational lesbian mothers who are actively involved throughout pregnancy report stronger attachment to babies after birth and better co-parenting relationships (Goldberg, 2006). Involvement during pregnancy matters for long-term family dynamics.

14.2 Attending Appointments Together

Both parents should attend prenatal appointments whenever possible. This signals to providers that you're both parents and helps the non-gestational partner stay connected.

Making appointments work for both:

Schedule strategically: Try to schedule appointments when both partners can attend. Some providers offer early morning, evening, or weekend appointments to accommodate work schedules.

Prioritize certain appointments: If you can't attend everything, prioritize ultrasounds (especially anatomy scan), first prenatal visit, and any appointments where major decisions will be made.

Virtual attendance: Some providers allow partners to join appointments virtually if they can't be physically present. This isn't ideal but better than missing entirely.

How non-gestational partners should engage at appointments:

Ask questions: Don't defer entirely to your pregnant partner. Ask your own questions about what's happening, what to expect, how to support.

Take notes: Write down important information so both of you retain what was discussed.

Advocate: If providers ignore you or direct everything to your pregnant partner, speak up: "I'm also a parent to this baby. Can you include me in this discussion?"

Be present: Put away your phone. Listen actively. Engage with what's happening. Your presence matters.

14.3 Managing External Perceptions

People often assume non-gestational partners are less important—support people rather than actual parents. This is wrong and damaging.

Common problematic assumptions:

- Medical staff directing all questions to pregnant person

- People referring to only the pregnant person as "parent" or "mother"
- Assuming non-gestational partner's role is just to support, not to parent
- Gendering partners incorrectly (calling lesbian non-gestational mothers "dad" or assuming they're just friends)
- Excluding non-gestational partners from conversations about baby care, feeding, parenting decisions

Correcting assumptions:

Be explicit: "We're both mothers to this baby." "I'm a parent too—please include me in this discussion." "I use she/her pronouns and I'm the non-gestational mother."

Visual cues: Both partners wearing wedding rings, holding hands, referring to each other as wives/partners/spouses signals relationship status.

Repetition: You'll need to correct people repeatedly. It's exhausting, but establishing that you're both parents from the beginning matters.

Provider preparation: Tell your prenatal care provider explicitly at the first appointment: "We're both parents to this baby. Both of us should receive medical information, participate in decisions, and be treated as equal parents. Please ensure your entire staff understands this."

14.4 Decision-Making as Co-Parents

Major decisions during pregnancy should involve both parents (or all parents in multi-parent families), not just the pregnant person.

Decisions requiring co-parent input:

- Whether to do prenatal testing and which tests
- Whether to learn baby's sex
- Choosing a name

- Circumcision (if applicable)
- Feeding plans (chest/breastfeeding, formula, both)
- Who will be present at birth
- Whether to bank cord blood
- Where to give birth (home, birth center, hospital)
- Pediatrician selection
- Childcare plans
- Parental leave arrangements

Decision-making process:

Discuss early: Don't wait until you're forced to decide. Talk through potential decisions well before they become urgent.

Both do research: Don't rely entirely on the pregnant person to research and then report. Both partners should learn about options and share what you discover.

Respect disagreement: Sometimes you'll disagree. Work through disagreement respectfully—listening, compromising, finding solutions that both can accept.

Some decisions are pregnant person's: While most decisions should be shared, some legitimately belong to the pregnant person—epidural or unmedicated birth, for instance. Non-gestational partners can have opinions but ultimate decision rests with the person doing the labor.

14.5 When Both Want to Carry

In lesbian couples where both partners have uteruses, both might want the pregnancy experience. This requires negotiation and planning.

Options:

Take turns: One partner carries the first child, the other carries subsequent children. This allows both to experience pregnancy but not simultaneously.

Reciprocal IVF: One partner provides eggs, the other carries. Then for a second child, reverse roles. This gives both genetic and gestational connection across multiple children.

Accept one partner carrying all: Sometimes one partner wants pregnancy more intensely, or practical factors (age, career, health) make one person the logical choice for carrying. This requires the other partner to grieve not having the pregnancy experience while fully embracing parenthood.

Managing feelings if one carries all:

For the pregnant partner: Recognize your partner might have complex feelings about not carrying. Include them actively throughout pregnancy. Don't take their presence for granted.

For the non-pregnant partner: Your feelings of loss or envy are valid. You can grieve not experiencing pregnancy while celebrating your partner's pregnancy. Both emotions coexist. Consider therapy to process complex feelings.

Research shows lesbian couples who explicitly discuss and resolve who carries report better relationship satisfaction than couples who avoid the conversation or assume one person should carry without discussion (Chabot & Ames, 2004).

14.6 Supporting Your Pregnant Partner

Practical and emotional support from partners significantly affects pregnant people's experiences and mental health (Stapleton et al., 2012).

Physical support:

- Take over physical tasks as pregnancy progresses (housework, shopping, cooking)
- Provide massages, foot rubs, back support
- Help with tasks they can no longer do comfortably (tying shoes, reaching items, heavy lifting)
- Make food runs when cravings hit or nausea limits what they can tolerate
- Handle pet care, childcare for existing children, or other responsibilities

Emotional support:

- Listen without trying to fix every problem
- Validate difficult symptoms ("I know you're exhausted and everything hurts—that's real and hard")
- Celebrate milestones (first heartbeat, movement, passing each trimester)
- Check in regularly about how they're feeling emotionally, not just physically
- Be patient with mood swings and emotional intensity

Medical support:

- Attend appointments
- Remember information from appointments and help make decisions
- Advocate with providers if necessary
- Research options for prenatal testing, birth plans, pediatricians
- Help track symptoms, medications, questions for providers

Specific support for LGBTQ+ partners:

- Correct pronouns and family structure with medical staff
- Advocate against discrimination or microaggressions
- Validate feelings about being pregnant while LGBTQ+ (especially for transgender partners managing dysphoria)
- Buffer against ignorant comments from others

- Celebrate your unique family structure rather than treating it as something to endure

14.7 Managing Difficult Emotions

Non-gestational partners sometimes experience unexpected difficult emotions during pregnancy: jealousy, feeling left out, anxiety about parenthood, resentment, fear.

Common difficult emotions:

Jealousy: If you wanted to carry but your partner is carrying, watching them experience pregnancy might trigger jealousy. This is normal and doesn't mean you're not excited about the baby.

Feeling secondary: Medical systems, family, and friends often treat non-gestational partners as less important. This feels awful and might create resentment.

Fear: You're about to become a parent to a baby you didn't carry. That's scary. You might worry about bonding, about whether you'll feel like a "real" parent, about managing parenting responsibilities.

Resentment: Your partner gets sympathy, attention, and accommodations because they're pregnant. You're expected to just handle everything without complaint. This can breed resentment, especially if your partner doesn't acknowledge your support.

How to manage:

Acknowledge feelings: Don't suppress difficult emotions. Name them. "I feel jealous watching you experience pregnancy even though I'm excited about our baby." Acknowledging feelings reduces their power.

Communicate with partner: Tell your partner what you're feeling. They might not realize you're struggling. Good communication prevents resentment from building.

Therapy: Consider individual or couples therapy to process complex emotions. Therapists who specialize in LGBTQ+ families and reproductive issues can help.

Community: Connect with other non-gestational partners in LGBTQ+ families. Online communities exist specifically for non-gestational lesbian mothers, partners of transgender pregnant people, and other configurations. You're not alone in feeling this way.

Self-compassion: Be gentle with yourself. Having complex feelings doesn't make you a bad partner or parent. It makes you human.

14.8 Preparing Siblings

If you have existing children, they need preparation for a new sibling. This applies to children from previous relationships, adopted children, or biological children from previous pregnancies.

Age-appropriate preparation:

Toddlers (1-3 years): Keep explanations simple. "There's a baby growing in parent's belly. The baby will come live with us soon." Read books about new siblings. Let them see ultrasound pictures.

Preschoolers (3-5 years): More detailed explanations work. "The baby is growing inside [parent]. In about [timeframe], the baby will be born and become part of our family." Involve them in preparation—setting up nursery, shopping for baby items. Validate that a new baby will change things.

School-age children (6-12 years): They can understand pregnancy in more detail. Involve them in planning. Let them feel baby move. Discuss how family dynamics will change. Address concerns directly.

Teenagers: Include them in real conversations about how a new baby will affect family life. Discuss logistics, expectations, and their role (not responsible for childcare unless they volunteer).

Common sibling concerns:

- Will you still love me when the baby comes?
- Will the baby take my toys/room/stuff?
- Why does the baby get so much attention?
- Will I have to babysit?

Address concerns directly: Reassure that love isn't finite, that their space and belongings will be respected, that they're not responsible for childcare (though helping is appreciated), and that while baby will need lots of attention initially, you still love them just as much.

For LGBTQ+ families specifically: If existing children are from previous relationships or different family configurations, help them understand how the new baby fits into your family. "This baby will be your sibling. We're all family together."

14.9 Partner Example

Consider Nicole's experience (composite): Her wife Priya was pregnant with their first child. Nicole attended every appointment, felt every kick she could, talked to the baby constantly. But she struggled with feeling invisible—providers directed everything to Priya, strangers congratulated only Priya, family asked how "mom" was doing while Nicole stood right there.

At week 28, Nicole broke down crying. "I feel like I'm just a support person, not a parent." Priya hugged her and said, "You're absolutely a parent. We're both mothers. Let's make sure everyone knows it."

They started explicitly correcting people: "We're both mothers." They told the midwife they wanted all information directed to both of them. Nicole started answering questions even when directed to Priya: "We're planning to..." not "She's planning to..."

During labor, Nicole was actively involved—providing counterpressure, reminding Priya to breathe, advocating with medical staff. When their daughter was born, Nicole held her second (after Priya's immediate skin-to-skin) and introduced herself: "Hi baby girl, I'm your other mama. We've been waiting for you."

Nicole bottle-fed while Priya breastfed, ensuring she had equal feeding time with their daughter. Within weeks, their daughter clearly recognized both mothers, reaching for Nicole as readily as for Priya. By six months, Nicole couldn't remember feeling invisible—she was undeniably, obviously, completely a parent.

14.10 Core Partnership Principles

Non-gestational partners in LGBTQ+ families need active involvement throughout pregnancy to bond with the baby and be recognized as equal parents. Attending appointments, feeling movement, participating in preparation, and learning about fetal development all create connection. Medical systems often erase non-gestational partners, requiring persistent advocacy and correction.

Decision-making during pregnancy should involve all parents, not just the pregnant person. Both partners need to research options and discuss decisions together. When both want to carry, negotiation and planning matter. Supporting your pregnant partner physically, emotionally, and practically strengthens your relationship and their pregnancy experience.

Difficult emotions like jealousy, feeling secondary, and fear are normal for non-gestational partners. Acknowledging feelings, communicating openly, and seeking support helps manage them. Preparing existing children for a new sibling requires age-appropriate conversations and validation of concerns.

Active, involved, equal partnership during pregnancy creates foundation for equal parenting after birth.

Chapter 15.0: Prenatal Mental Health

Riley hit week 24 and couldn't stop crying. Everything triggered tears—commercials, dropped forks, the thought of becoming a parent. They'd struggled with anxiety for years, but pregnancy made it worse. Plus, as a non-binary person with a growing belly, dysphoria was constant. Strangers gendered them as female everywhere they went. They felt trapped in a body they didn't recognize, anxious about parenthood, and completely overwhelmed.

Prenatal mental health matters. Pregnancy hormones affect mood. The vulnerability of pregnancy triggers anxiety. For LGBTQ+ people, pregnancy often brings additional stressors: dysphoria, discrimination, isolation, and fear. This chapter covers common emotional challenges in LGBTQ+ pregnancy, dysphoria management, dealing with discrimination, building resilience, when to seek help, medication safety, and finding community.

15.1 Common Emotional Challenges

Pregnancy affects mental health even for people without pre-existing mental health conditions. Hormones fluctuate. Your body changes dramatically. You're facing massive life transition. And LGBTQ+ people experience additional layers of challenge.

Anxiety: About 15-20% of pregnant people experience significant anxiety during pregnancy (Goodman et al., 2016). Worry about miscarriage, baby's health, labor, ability to parent, finances, relationship stability—all common. For LGBTQ+ people, add worries about discrimination, whether family will accept your baby, legal protection of parental rights, and managing your identity while pregnant.

Depression: About 10-15% of pregnant people experience depression during pregnancy, often called **perinatal depression** (American College of Obstetricians and Gynecologists, 2023). Symptoms include persistent sadness, loss of interest in activities, difficulty concentrating, changes in sleep or appetite, feelings of worthlessness or hopelessness. This is different from occasional pregnancy mood swings—it's persistent and interferes with functioning.

Mood swings: Hormonal fluctuations cause rapid emotional shifts. You cry over nothing. You snap at your partner. You feel euphoric then devastated within hours. This is normal in pregnancy, though exhausting.

Fear of labor: Nearly everyone fears labor to some degree. It's painful, unpredictable, and involves loss of control. For LGBTQ+ people, fear might include being misgendered during labor, discrimination from hospital staff, or (for transgender and non-binary people) dysphoria during intimate medical procedures.

Fear of parenthood: The enormity of becoming responsible for a helpless human terrifies most people. For LGBTQ+ parents, additional fears might include whether you'll bond adequately (especially for non-gestational parents), how to protect your child from discrimination, whether you'll be good enough parents despite lacking models of LGBTQ+ parenthood.

Isolation: Pregnancy can be isolating for anyone. For LGBTQ+ people, isolation intensifies if you don't know other LGBTQ+ parents, if family isn't supportive, or if pregnancy spaces feel unwelcoming due to gendered language and heteronormative assumptions.

15.2 Dysphoria Throughout Pregnancy

For transgender men and non-binary pregnant people, dysphoria often intensifies as pregnancy progresses and body changes become more pronounced.

Dysphoria triggers:

- Growing belly making pregnancy visible
- Breast/chest development
- Being constantly gendered as female by strangers
- Inability to bind
- Wearing maternity clothes designed for women
- Prenatal care involving pelvic exams and intimate examinations
- Feeling trapped in an increasingly feminine-appearing body

Wave-like pattern: Many transgender and non-binary pregnant people report that dysphoria comes in waves—some days or weeks are manageable, others are horrible. First trimester is often hard, second trimester sometimes improves as you focus on baby rather than symptoms, third trimester is often hardest as visibility peaks.

Management strategies (expanding on what we covered in Chapter 13.0):

Reframing: Find mental frameworks that reduce dysphoria's impact. Some people view pregnancy as an inherently masculine experience for men with uteruses. Others separate "my identity" from "what my body is doing temporarily." Find what works for you.

Control what you can: Choose your own language (chest not breasts, they/them not she/her). Wear clothes that feel authentic. Limit exposure to triggering content.

Therapy: Work with a therapist who understands transgender identity and pregnancy. Having professional support for processing dysphoria matters enormously.

Community: Connect with other transgender and non-binary pregnant people or parents. Online communities exist specifically for this. Knowing others have done this successfully reduces isolation.

Endpoint focus: Remember this is temporary. You will give birth. You will resume testosterone if that's your plan. You will return to your chest binder or pursue top surgery. Pregnancy has an endpoint.

15.3 Discrimination and Microaggressions

LGBTQ+ people experience discrimination and microaggressions throughout pregnancy in healthcare settings, social situations, and public spaces.

Common microaggressions:

- "Where's dad?" asked to lesbian mothers
- "So who's the real mom?" asked to two mothers
- Pronoun mistakes despite corrections
- Assuming non-gestational partners are friends or support people rather than parents
- "You're pregnant?!" with surprise and confusion directed at transgender men
- Invasive questions about conception ("So how did you...?")
- Comments suggesting LGBTQ+ people shouldn't have children
- Religious-based judgment or attempts to convert

Impact on mental health: Discrimination and microaggressions cause stress, anxiety, and trauma. Repeated small aggressions accumulate into significant psychological burden. For people already managing pregnancy anxiety or dysphoria, discrimination adds overwhelming additional stress (Velez et al., 2021).

Coping strategies:

Prepared responses: Have scripts ready for common microaggressions:

- "We're both mothers to this baby."
- "Yes, transgender men can get pregnant."
- "How we conceived is private information."

- "I use he/him pronouns."

Selective disclosure: You don't owe everyone your story. Share what feels safe and skip details with strangers or unsafe people.

Build support team: Surround yourself with affirming people who validate your experience and buffer against discrimination.

Report serious discrimination: If healthcare providers discriminate, report to patient advocates, medical boards, or legal organizations like Lambda Legal. You don't have to accept mistreatment.

Therapy: Process discrimination-related trauma with a therapist. Don't minimize its impact.

15.4 Building Resilience

Resilience—the ability to adapt and bounce back from adversity—protects mental health during stressful periods like pregnancy.

Strategies for building resilience:

Self-advocacy: Practice speaking up for your needs, correcting mistakes, and setting boundaries. The more you advocate successfully, the more confident you become.

Support network: Build strong connections with affirming people—partners, friends, chosen family, LGBTQ+ community, online support groups. Social support is one of the strongest predictors of resilience.

Self-care: Prioritize sleep, nutrition, movement, and activities that restore you. Self-care isn't selfish during pregnancy—it's necessary.

Mindfulness: Practices like meditation, deep breathing, or mindfulness apps can reduce stress and improve emotional regulation. Even five minutes daily helps.

Realistic expectations: Don't expect yourself to handle everything perfectly. Pregnancy is hard. Being LGBTQ+ adds complexity. Give yourself permission to struggle sometimes.

Celebrate wins: Notice when things go well—a good prenatal appointment, a provider who gets your pronouns right, feeling baby move, making it through a difficult week. Celebrate these moments rather than only focusing on what's hard.

15.5 When to Seek Help

Knowing when typical pregnancy emotions cross into clinical mental health concerns requiring professional help matters.

Signs you need professional support:

- Persistent sadness or hopelessness lasting more than two weeks
- Loss of interest in activities you normally enjoy
- Difficulty functioning in daily life (work, relationships, self-care)
- Thoughts of harming yourself
- Panic attacks or severe anxiety interfering with life
- Obsessive thoughts or compulsive behaviors
- Trauma symptoms (flashbacks, nightmares, hypervigilance)
- Dysphoria so severe you can't function
- Substance use to cope with emotions

Don't wait: If you're struggling, seek help early. Mental health problems during pregnancy don't resolve on their own and often worsen without treatment. Early intervention prevents escalation.

Who to contact:

- Your prenatal care provider (they can screen for mental health concerns and refer you)
- A therapist specializing in perinatal mental health and ideally LGBTQ+ competency

- Psychiatrist for medication evaluation if needed
- Postpartum Support International warmline: 1-800-944-4773
- Crisis lines if you're in immediate distress (988 Suicide and Crisis Lifeline)

15.6 Medications and Therapy

Some pregnant people need mental health medications. Many medications are safe during pregnancy, and untreated mental health conditions often pose greater risks than medication does.

Therapy during pregnancy: Psychotherapy is first-line treatment for mild to moderate prenatal anxiety and depression. Cognitive-behavioral therapy (CBT) and interpersonal therapy (IPT) have strong evidence for treating perinatal mental health conditions (Sockol, 2015).

Look for therapists who:

- Specialize in perinatal mental health
- Have LGBTQ+ competency and ideally specific experience with LGBTQ+ pregnancy
- Use evidence-based approaches (CBT, IPT, DBT, ACT)
- Are available regularly (weekly sessions often work best)

Medications during pregnancy: If therapy alone isn't sufficient, or if you have moderate to severe mental health conditions, medication might be necessary.

Safe medications: Many psychiatric medications have good safety data in pregnancy:

- Certain SSRIs (sertraline, fluoxetine) are commonly prescribed for depression and anxiety
- Some anxiety medications are safe (though benzodiazepines are generally avoided)
- Mood stabilizers vary in safety—work with a psychiatrist to find options

Risk assessment: All medications carry some risk. So does untreated mental health condition. The question isn't "Is this medication completely risk-free?" (nothing is) but rather "Do benefits outweigh risks?" Work with a psychiatrist who specializes in perinatal mental health to make informed decisions.

Don't stop medications without consulting your provider: If you were taking psychiatric medications before pregnancy, don't stop suddenly. Work with your prescriber to evaluate whether continuing, switching, or carefully discontinuing makes sense for your situation.

15.7 Community Connection

Finding community significantly improves mental health during pregnancy for LGBTQ+ people.

LGBTQ+ parenting communities:

- Local LGBTQ+ parenting groups (check Pride centers, PFLAG chapters, community centers)
- Online forums and social media groups for LGBTQ+ pregnancy and parenting
- Specific communities for transgender pregnancy, lesbian mothers, non-binary parents, etc.

General pregnancy communities (with caveats): Regular pregnancy groups provide practical information but might not feel inclusive. Join selectively and leave if gendered language triggers dysphoria or heteronormative assumptions feel alienating.

Mental health support groups: Perinatal mental health support groups exist in many areas, often run through hospitals or community mental health centers. These provide peer support specifically for pregnancy-related mental health challenges.

Benefits of community: Connection with others having similar experiences reduces isolation, provides practical advice, normalizes struggles, offers hope, and creates lasting friendships. Many LGBTQ+ parents report that friendships formed during pregnancy and early parenthood become central to their support networks for years.

15.8 Composite Example

Consider Alex and Riley's mental health journey (composite): Riley, a non-binary person carrying their first pregnancy, struggled with anxiety throughout. By week 20, they were having panic attacks several times a week, catastrophizing about labor, obsessing over whether the baby was okay, and barely sleeping.

Alex, their wife, encouraged Riley to talk to their midwife. The midwife screened Riley for anxiety and referred them to a perinatal mental health therapist. Riley started weekly therapy using cognitive-behavioral approaches to manage anxiety.

The therapist taught Riley breathing techniques, helped them identify catastrophic thinking patterns and challenge them, and worked on building distress tolerance. Riley also joined an online support group for LGBTQ+ pregnancy where they connected with other non-binary and transgender pregnant people.

By week 32, Riley's panic attacks had decreased significantly. They still felt anxious sometimes—pregnancy is inherently anxiety-provoking—but they had tools to manage it. They continued therapy through pregnancy and postpartum, preventing postpartum anxiety from overwhelming them.

Looking back, Riley said: "I almost didn't get help because I thought pregnancy anxiety was normal and I should just tough it out. Getting therapy was the best decision I made during pregnancy."

15.9 Essential Mental Health Points

Prenatal mental health matters for healthy pregnancy experiences and long-term wellbeing. Anxiety, depression, mood swings, fear, and isolation are common during pregnancy, with LGBTQ+ people experiencing additional stressors including dysphoria, discrimination, and lack of community.

Dysphoria often intensifies during pregnancy for transgender and non-binary people, requiring active management through reframing, therapy, community support, and focusing on pregnancy's temporary nature. Discrimination and microaggressions cause significant psychological harm—building resilience, using prepared responses, and reporting serious discrimination helps manage this.

Seek professional help when struggling—don't wait for mental health problems to resolve on their own. Therapy and medications are both evidence-based treatments for prenatal mental health conditions. Many medications are safe during pregnancy when needed. Finding LGBTQ+ community reduces isolation and provides peer support.

Taking care of your mental health during pregnancy isn't optional or selfish—it's necessary for your wellbeing and your baby's wellbeing. Ask for help when you need it.

Part Four: Birth Preparation and Labor

Chapter 16.0: Creating Birth Preferences

Isabella and Carmen spent weeks crafting their birth plan. They wanted their document to communicate clearly: Carmen was as much a mother as Isabella, they both needed to be included in all decisions, and staff should use "mothers" plural when referring to them. They specified who would cut the cord (Carmen), that they both wanted immediate skin-to-skin time, and that they were open to pain management but wanted to avoid unnecessary interventions.

The birth plan worked. When they arrived in labor, nurses read it and immediately understood their family structure. Throughout labor, staff directed questions to both of them and respected their preferences. Having spent time thinking through and articulating what mattered made their birth experience significantly better than it would have been otherwise.

Creating birth preferences (commonly called a birth plan) involves thinking through what matters to you during labor and birth, communicating that to your care team, and preparing for the reality that labor doesn't always go as planned. This chapter covers components of inclusive birth preferences, language considerations, pain management, who will be present, immediate postpartum preferences, feeding plans, newborn procedures, and LGBTQ+ specific considerations.

16.1 What Birth Preferences Include

Birth preferences communicate your hopes and priorities for labor, birth, and immediate postpartum to your care team. They're not binding contracts—labor can't be fully controlled—but they guide decision-making.

Key components:

- Your identity, family structure, and language preferences
- Pain management approach
- Movement and positioning preferences
- Interventions you want to avoid unless necessary
- Who will be present
- Immediate postpartum preferences (skin-to-skin, cord clamping, etc.)
- Feeding plans
- Newborn procedures (vitamin K, eye ointment, hepatitis B vaccine, circumcision)

Format: One to two pages maximum. Bullet points or short paragraphs. Readable at a glance. Providers and nurses are busy during labor—make it easy for them to understand quickly what matters to you.

16.2 Language Considerations

For LGBTQ+ families, language in birth preferences matters enormously because it sets expectations about how staff should address you and your family.

What to specify:

Pronouns: "I use he/him pronouns." "I use they/them pronouns." "We both use she/her pronouns." State this prominently at the beginning.

Partner titles: "My wife is my baby's other mother." "My husband is supporting me during labor—he's not the baby's father." "We're both mothers to this baby." "I'm the father, not the mother, despite being pregnant."

Anatomy terms: If you have preferences about anatomy language, state them: "Please refer to my chest rather than breasts." "Use neutral anatomy terms when possible." Most providers will use standard medical terms unless you specify otherwise.

Family terms: How you want staff to refer to your family: "Please use 'mothers' plural when discussing parents." "I'm a father, not a mother." "Both parents should receive all medical information."

Example language section from birth plan:

"I'm Marcus (he/him), a transgender man having my first baby. My spouse is Tao (he/him). I'm the father, not the mother. Please use he/him pronouns and masculine language when referring to me. Use neutral terms like 'chest' rather than 'breasts.' Both Tao and I are this baby's fathers."

Or:

"I'm Riley (they/them), a non-binary person. My wife is Alex (she/her). Please use they/them pronouns for me and gender-neutral language. We're both parents to this baby. Alex is a mother; I prefer the term 'parent' or 'ren' rather than mother or father."

16.3 Pain Management Options

Pain management is deeply personal. Some people want unmedicated birth. Others want epidurals. Many want to see how labor goes before deciding. All approaches are valid.

Unmedicated birth: Using non-pharmacological comfort measures (movement, positioning, breathing, water, massage, hypnosis, visualization). Benefits include mobility, avoiding medication side effects, and some people find it empowering. Challenges include that labor is extremely painful and managing intense pain requires significant physical and mental work.

Epidural analgesia: Medication inserted through catheter into the epidural space of your spine that numbs the lower body. Benefits include very effective pain relief, ability to rest during long labor.

Challenges include restricted mobility (you're in bed once epidural is placed), potential for slowing labor, rare side effects, and interventions cascade (epidural often requires continuous monitoring, IV fluids, urinary catheter).

Nitrous oxide (where available): Inhaled gas that reduces pain perception without eliminating it. Benefits include staying mobile and alert, no major side effects, you control when you use it. Challenges include that it only dulls pain (doesn't eliminate it) and causes nausea for some people.

IV pain medications (opioids): Medications given through IV that reduce pain. Benefits include pain relief without epidural restrictions. Challenges include drowsiness, nausea, can cross placenta affecting baby, less effective than epidural.

State your approach in birth preferences:

If you want unmedicated: "I'm planning unmedicated birth using movement, positioning, breathing, and water for comfort. Please don't offer pain medications unless I request them."

If you want epidural: "I'm planning to use epidural analgesia. Please let me know when epidural placement is available."

If you're deciding in the moment: "I'm undecided about pain management. I'll assess during labor and request what I need. Please provide information about options but let me initiate conversations about pain relief."

16.4 Who Will Be Present

Decide who you want present during labor and birth, and specify their roles in your birth preferences.

Support people:

- Partner/spouse

- Doula
- Close friends or family
- Multiple support people if your birth setting allows

Roles: Specify what each person will do. For LGBTQ+ families, be explicit about partner roles: "My wife Carmen will be actively supporting me throughout labor. She will cut the cord and have immediate skin-to-skin time with our baby. She is a mother to this baby, not just a support person."

Partner considerations for LGBTQ+ families:

Both parents present: If you have two parents, specify that both should be present and involved. Hospitals sometimes have policies limiting support people, but legal parents (or soon-to-be-legal parents) should be allowed.

Correct gendering: "My partner uses she/her pronouns and is the baby's other mother." State this clearly so staff don't misgender partners based on appearance.

Equal information: "All medical information should be provided to both of us. We're both parents and both make decisions."

Photography and video: Specify if you want someone taking photos or video, and any restrictions (no photos during actual delivery, for instance).

16.5 Immediate Postpartum Preferences

The hour after birth significantly affects bonding, breastfeeding initiation, and overall birth experience.

Delayed cord clamping: Waiting to clamp and cut the umbilical cord (typically 1-3 minutes after birth) allows more blood to transfer from placenta to baby. Research shows benefits for baby's iron stores and potentially other health outcomes (McDonald et al.,

2013). Most providers now recommend this unless emergency requires immediate cord cutting.

Skin-to-skin: Placing baby directly on your chest immediately after birth (before weighing, measuring, or bathing). This helps regulate baby's temperature, heart rate, and breathing, supports bonding, and facilitates breastfeeding initiation. Most providers now recommend immediate skin-to-skin for at least an hour.

For LGBTQ+ families with two parents: Specify who gets first skin-to-skin (typically the gestational parent) and when the second parent gets skin-to-skin time. "I want immediate skin-to-skin. After about 30 minutes, my wife would like skin-to-skin time with our baby."

For transgender men: Skin-to-skin might trigger dysphoria. Specify what you want: "I want brief skin-to-skin while the cord is being cut, then my partner will hold the baby." Or: "I prefer my partner to have first skin-to-skin time. I'll hold the baby while clothed or wrapped in a blanket."

Newborn procedures: Specify timing for routine procedures:

- "Please delay weighing and measuring until after the first hour of skin-to-skin and first feeding attempt."
- "No routine bath for at least 24 hours."
- "All procedures that don't require separation can happen while baby is on my chest."

16.6 Feeding Plans

State your feeding intentions in birth preferences so staff know how to support you.

If chest/breastfeeding: "I plan to chest-feed. I'd like support with latching during the first hour after birth. No pacifiers or bottles unless medically necessary."

If formula feeding: "We're planning to formula feed. Please provide formula and bottles."

If combination feeding: "We're planning to combine chest/breastfeeding and formula feeding. Please support both."

For non-gestational parents: "Both parents will be feeding the baby. [Non-gestational parent] will be giving bottles."

For transgender men: Specify if you're chest-feeding and what language you want used: "I plan to chest-feed. Please use the term 'chest-feeding' rather than breastfeeding." Or: "I won't be chest-feeding. Please provide formula."

16.7 Newborn Procedures

Several routine newborn procedures occur in the first 24 hours. You consent or decline for each.

Vitamin K injection: Recommended to prevent vitamin K deficiency bleeding. Most providers strongly recommend this. Research supports safety and benefit.

Erythromycin eye ointment: Applied to prevent eye infections from bacteria baby might encounter during birth. Some parents decline this if they were screened for STIs during pregnancy and are confident of no exposure.

Hepatitis B vaccine: First dose of hepatitis B vaccine is typically given in the hospital. Many parents consent. Some prefer to delay until later pediatrician visits.

Circumcision (if baby is assigned male at birth): This is a personal decision based on cultural, religious, medical, or aesthetic preferences. There's no universal recommendation. If you plan circumcision, it typically happens before hospital discharge (for hospital births) or within the first few weeks.

State your preferences clearly: "Please give vitamin K injection and hepatitis B vaccine. We decline eye ointment as we were screened for STIs. If the baby is male, we haven't decided about circumcision yet—please don't perform it without discussing with us first."

16.8 LGBTQ+ Specific Considerations

Include explicit statements in birth preferences about your identity, family structure, and how staff should interact with you.

Identity statement: Open with who you are and your family structure: "We're Isabella and Carmen, a lesbian couple having our first baby together. Isabella is carrying, and we're both mothers."

Equal treatment: "Both mothers should be included in all medical discussions and decisions. Please direct information to both of us, not only to Isabella."

Language policing: "Please use she/her pronouns for both of us and refer to us as 'mothers' plural. If you hear staff using incorrect language, please correct them."

Discrimination response plan: "If we experience discrimination or misgendering, we will contact patient advocates immediately. Please help us ensure respectful care."

Partner rights: "Carmen has full rights to make medical decisions if Isabella is unable to. She should be present for all procedures and should remain with the baby if separation from Isabella is necessary."

Legal documentation: If you've already completed legal steps establishing parental rights, note this: "We're legally married. Second-parent adoption paperwork has been initiated." This sometimes helps staff understand your family structure is legally recognized.

16.9 Flexibility and Reality

Include a statement acknowledging that birth doesn't always go as planned:

"These preferences represent our hopes for an uncomplicated birth. We understand that circumstances sometimes require changes to plans. If interventions become medically necessary, please explain why and discuss options with both of us. We trust our medical team to help us make informed decisions while respecting our preferences as much as possible."

This signals that you're reasonable and understand birth's unpredictability while maintaining that your preferences matter.

16.10 Sample Framework

Here's a framework for an inclusive birth plan:

BIRTH PREFERENCES FOR [YOUR NAMES]

About Our Family: [Brief statement about who you are, pronouns, partner relationships, any specific language needs]

Pain Management: [Your approach—unmedicated, epidural, deciding in labor, etc.]

Movement and Positioning: [Preferences about staying mobile, trying various positions, using birth tools like balls or tubs]

Support People: [Who will be present and their roles, emphasizing partner's parental status]

Interventions: [What you want to avoid unless necessary—continuous monitoring, IV, artificial rupture of membranes, etc.]

Birth: [Preferences for pushing, positions, who catches baby or cuts cord]

Immediate Postpartum: [Skin-to-skin, delayed cord clamping, when newborn procedures happen]

Feeding: [Your feeding plan]

Newborn Procedures: [Consent or decline for vitamin K, eye ointment, hepatitis B vaccine, circumcision]

If Cesarean Becomes Necessary: [Preferences for gentle cesarean—partner present, see baby immediately, skin-to-skin in OR if possible]

Final Note: [Statement about flexibility and trust in your care team]

16.11 Key Planning Insights

Birth preferences communicate your hopes for labor, birth, and immediate postpartum while acknowledging birth's unpredictability. For LGBTQ+ families, birth preferences explicitly state identity, pronouns, family structure, and language needs, ensuring staff understand how to address you respectfully.

Include preferences for pain management, movement, who's present, immediate postpartum, feeding, and newborn procedures. Keep the document brief (1-2 pages), readable, and realistic. Bring multiple copies to give each shift of nurses and providers.

Good birth preferences balance expressing what matters to you with acknowledging that medical circumstances sometimes require flexibility. They're conversation starters with your care team, not rigid demands. The goal is informed, respectful, collaborative decision-making throughout labor and birth.

Chapter 17.0: Preparing Hospitals and Birth Centers

Two weeks before Isabella's due date, she and Carmen met with the hospital's patient advocate. They brought copies of their birth plan, explained their family structure, and walked through what they needed: both mothers treated equally, correct pronouns consistently, no assumptions about family structure, equal access to baby during and after birth. The patient advocate took notes, added flags to Isabella's chart, and committed to briefing labor and delivery staff about inclusive care.

When Isabella went into labor at 39 weeks, the preparation paid off. The intake nurse saw the notes and immediately used correct language. The labor nurse read their birth plan and addressed both of them as mothers throughout. When problems arose requiring conversation with an obstetrician, that doctor consulted both of them. The experience wasn't perfect—one nurse kept defaulting to "mom" singular until corrected—but overall, the advance preparation created significantly better care than they would have received otherwise.

This chapter covers preparing hospitals or birth centers for LGBTQ+ families: communicating needs in advance, working with patient advocates, training staff, documentation considerations, room assignments, preparing for potential discrimination, and backup plans.

17.1 Communicating Needs in Advance

Don't wait until you're in labor to tell the hospital about your family structure and needs. Advance communication prepares staff and reduces likelihood of problems.

When to reach out: Around 34-36 weeks, contact the hospital or birth center where you plan to give birth. Ask to meet with a patient advocate, social worker, or nurse manager to discuss your needs.

What to communicate:

- Your identity and pronouns
- Your partner's identity and parental status
- Language preferences (what terms you want used)
- Family structure (both mothers, father giving birth, non-binary parent, three parents, etc.)
- Any specific concerns about discrimination or past negative experiences
- Request that staff be informed about your family before you arrive in labor

How to communicate: Schedule an in-person or phone meeting. Bring written information (your birth plan, a brief letter explaining your family, documentation of legal marriage or parental status if relevant). Follow up via email documenting what was discussed.

Example language: "Hi, I'm scheduled to give birth at your hospital in about four weeks. I'm a transgender man, and I want to ensure your staff are prepared to provide respectful care. Can I meet with someone to discuss my needs and make sure appropriate documentation is in my chart?"

17.2 Working with Patient Advocates

Most hospitals have patient advocates or social workers whose job includes helping patients navigate the system and ensuring respectful care. Use them.

What patient advocates can do:

- Add notes to your chart about your identity, pronouns, family structure
- Brief labor and delivery staff about your family

- Provide education to staff who may not have worked with LGBTQ+ families
- Help resolve problems if discrimination occurs during labor
- Connect you with supportive resources within the hospital
- Advocate with administration if policies need adjustment

Preparing for the meeting:

- Bring your birth plan
- Explain your family structure clearly
- State specific concerns based on past experiences or fears
- Ask about hospital policies on partner presence, decision-making, legal parent recognition
- Request specific accommodations you need

Documentation in your chart: Ask the patient advocate to add visible notes to your chart that labor and delivery staff will see immediately: "Patient uses he/him pronouns—please use masculine language." "Two mothers—both are parents with equal decision-making authority." "Non-binary patient—use they/them pronouns and gender-neutral language."

17.3 Training Staff

Ideally, hospitals would train all staff on LGBTQ+ cultural competency before you arrive. In reality, many hospitals have minimal LGBTQ+ training. Your advance visit creates opportunity for education.

Offer to provide resources: If the hospital seems open but inexperienced, offer resources: "I can provide links to resources on transgender pregnancy if that would help your staff prepare."

Brief in-service education: Some hospitals will arrange brief in-service education for labor and delivery staff about LGBTQ+ families. This might be a 30-minute presentation or even just a memo. If they're willing, take advantage.

Your birth plan as education: Your birth plan itself educates staff. Clear, explicit language teaches them how to interact with you: "I'm Marcus, a transgender man (he/him pronouns). I'm the father, not the mother. My spouse Tao is also a father—we're both this baby's fathers."

Reality check: You can't fully train hospital staff before you arrive. Some education will happen during your labor. Prepare for this likelihood while hoping your advance work minimizes it.

17.4 Documentation and Wristbands

Hospital documentation systems often struggle with LGBTQ+ families because they're designed assuming heterosexual, cisgender patients.

Name on wristband: Your name band should display the name you actually use, not just your legal name if they differ. Fight for this if necessary—being called the wrong name repeatedly during labor is dehumanizing.

Gender marker: Wristbands might display gender. If your gender marker doesn't match your reproductive anatomy (common for transgender patients), this confuses staff. Some hospitals allow removing gender from wristbands or using neutral markers. Request this if it reduces misgendering.

Partner identification: Make sure your partner receives appropriate identification showing they're a parent. Some hospitals provide wristbands to partners that allow them to accompany baby to nursery, hold baby in NICU if needed, and make medical decisions.

Chart documentation: Your medical chart should reflect accurate information:

- Name and pronouns prominently displayed
- Partner listed as partner/spouse, not "support person"
- Both parents' names in relevant fields

- Notes about your family structure visible to all staff

Advocate if documentation is wrong: If you see incorrect information in your chart or on wristbands, request immediate correction. "This says 'mother' but I'm the father. Please change it." Don't let incorrect documentation stand.

17.5 Room Assignments

Where you give birth and recover matters for privacy, comfort, and partner accommodation.

Private room: Request a private room for labor, delivery, and postpartum recovery. This gives you more privacy and reduces exposure to potential discrimination from roommates or their visitors.

Partner accommodation: Confirm that your partner can stay overnight in your room after birth. Most hospitals allow this, but policies vary. For LGBTQ+ families, explicitly establish that your partner is a parent, not just a visitor.

Multiple partners: If you have more than two parents (polyamorous families, co-parenting arrangements), discuss how the hospital handles this. Visitor policies might limit numbers, but parents should be treated differently from visitors.

Bathroom access: If you're a transgender man or non-binary person, clarify which bathroom you should use. Some hospitals have single-stall or gender-neutral bathrooms. Don't accept being directed to a bathroom that doesn't match your gender identity.

17.6 Preparing for Discrimination

Despite best efforts, discrimination sometimes happens. Prepare backup plans.

Know your rights: You have the right to respectful care regardless of sexual orientation or gender identity. Federal protections exist, and many states have additional protections. Know this going in: mistreatment is not something you must tolerate.

Patient advocate contact info: Get the name and direct phone number of the patient advocate you met with. If problems arise during labor, your partner can call them immediately.

Escalation plan: Know who to contact if problems occur:

1. First: Ask to speak with charge nurse or nurse manager
2. Second: Contact patient advocate
3. Third: Request administrative supervisor
4. Fourth: File formal complaint after birth

Your partner as advocate: During labor, you'll be physically vulnerable and possibly not capable of advocating for yourself. Your partner's role includes advocating against discrimination—correcting pronouns, requesting different staff if someone is problematic, calling for help if needed.

Document everything: If discrimination occurs, write down names, times, what happened. This documentation supports formal complaints or legal action if necessary.

Lambda Legal and other resources: Organizations like Lambda Legal provide legal support for LGBTQ+ people experiencing healthcare discrimination. Know these resources exist if you need them.

17.7 Backup Plans

Sometimes despite preparation, a hospital or birth center proves unable or unwilling to provide respectful care. Have backup plans.

Alternative birth location: If you meet with a hospital and they're resistant or you don't feel safe, consider:

- Different hospital in your area
- Birth center if available
- Home birth if appropriate for your risk level

Different provider: If your provider practices at a problematic hospital, discuss whether they have privileges at alternative hospitals or whether you should switch providers.

Transfer plans: If you're planning birth center or home birth and transfer to hospital becomes necessary, communicate your needs to receiving hospital's staff immediately upon arrival. Your midwife or birth center staff can advocate for you.

Legal representation: In extreme cases where hospitals refuse to provide appropriate care or violate your rights, legal representation might be necessary. This is rare but possible. Contact LGBTQ+ legal organizations if you face serious discrimination.

17.8 Example of Successful Preparation

Consider Kai's experience (composite): At 34 weeks, Kai (a transgender man) and his husband Tao met with their hospital's patient advocate. Kai explained he was a trans man having his first baby, he used he/him pronouns, he was the father not the mother, and he was very concerned about being misgendered during labor when he'd be vulnerable.

The patient advocate was unfamiliar with transgender pregnancy but eager to learn. She added prominent notes to Kai's chart: "Patient is transgender man. Use HE/HIM pronouns and masculine language. Refer to 'chest' not 'breasts.' Patient's spouse Tao is also a father—both are this baby's fathers."

She emailed labor and delivery nursing staff with brief guidance on transgender pregnancy and Kai's specific needs. She gave Kai her cell phone number to call if any problems arose during labor.

When Kai arrived in labor at 39 weeks, the intake nurse saw the chart notes and immediately used correct pronouns. Throughout labor, nurses consistently called Kai "he" and referred to him as "dad." When one nurse slipped and said "mama," another nurse immediately corrected her.

Was it perfect? No. Kai still had moments of dysphoria and discomfort. But the respect was present in a way it wouldn't have been without advance preparation. The patient advocate called the day after delivery to check how it went. Kai's feedback helped the hospital improve their processes for future LGBTQ+ patients.

17.9 Birth Center Considerations

Birth centers are often more personalized and might provide more culturally competent care than large hospitals, but they vary.

Advantages of birth centers:

- Smaller staff teams you can meet in advance
- Often more progressive policies and practices
- Midwifery model of care typically more patient-centered
- Easier to ensure all staff know your family structure

Questions to ask birth centers:

- How many LGBTQ+ families have you served?
- How do you train staff on inclusive care?
- Can we meet all staff who might attend our birth?
- How do you handle documentation for LGBTQ+ families?
- What happens if we need to transfer to a hospital?

Transfer considerations: Birth centers handle low-risk births. If complications arise requiring hospital transfer, you'll arrive at a hospital mid-emergency. Make sure your birth plan and identity information go with you so receiving hospital staff have some preparation.

17.10 Final Preparation Checklist

Before your due date, complete these steps:

- [ ] Schedule meeting with hospital patient advocate or social worker (around week 34-36)
- [ ] Discuss your identity, family structure, pronouns, language needs
- [ ] Request notes be added to your chart that all staff will see
- [ ] Provide copies of birth plan to hospital for your chart
- [ ] Get patient advocate's direct contact information
- [ ] Confirm partner's rights—can they stay overnight, make decisions, access baby?
- [ ] Clarify room assignment preferences
- [ ] Discuss what happens if discrimination occurs
- [ ] Make sure your partner knows who to contact if problems arise
- [ ] Bring multiple copies of birth plan to labor (give fresh copy to each shift)
- [ ] Have backup plans ready if hospital proves problematic

Advance preparation doesn't guarantee perfect care, but it dramatically improves chances of respectful treatment during one of life's most vulnerable moments.

17.11 Core Preparation Principles

Preparing hospitals and birth centers for LGBTQ+ families requires advance communication, working with patient advocates, ensuring proper documentation, and having backup plans for discrimination. Meet with patient advocates or social workers around week 34-36 to explain your needs and request appropriate chart documentation.

Clear communication about identity, pronouns, family structure, and language needs prepares staff to provide respectful care. Documentation systems should reflect accurate names, pronouns, and family relationships. Private rooms and confirmed partner accommodations matter for comfort and privacy.

Know your rights and have escalation plans if discrimination occurs. Patient advocates, charge nurses, and administrative supervisors can address problems. Document any discrimination for formal complaints. In extreme cases, legal representation through organizations like Lambda Legal may be necessary.

Birth centers often provide more personalized care but transfer plans to hospitals are essential for complications. Advance preparation makes birth experiences significantly better for LGBTQ+ families, reducing stress and discrimination during labor and delivery.

Chapter 18.0: Labor and Birth Experiences

Elena's contractions started at 3am—mild cramping that woke her. By 6am, they were coming every ten minutes. By noon, every five minutes. By 6pm, she was in the hospital, dilated to 6 centimeters, working through intense contractions while Jasmine held her hand and reminded her to breathe. By 10pm, she was pushing. At 11:47pm, their daughter was born, screaming and perfect.

Labor is intense, unpredictable, and transformative. Understanding what happens during labor, how to cope with contractions, when to go to the hospital, and how partners can support effectively helps you approach birth with knowledge rather than fear. This chapter covers stages of labor, early labor management, active labor coping techniques, transition, pushing and birth, the midwifery model, partner support, and pain management options.

18.1 Stages of Labor

Labor progresses through distinct stages, though timing varies enormously between individuals and between first and subsequent births.

First stage (cervical dilation): From first regular contractions until cervix is fully dilated to 10 centimeters. This stage has three phases:

Early labor (0-6 cm dilation): Contractions are mild to moderate, typically 5-20 minutes apart, lasting 30-60 seconds each. This phase can last hours to days, especially for first babies. You can usually talk through early labor contractions.

Active labor (6-8 cm dilation): Contractions intensify—strong, regular, closer together (typically 3-5 minutes apart), lasting 60-90 seconds. You need to focus through contractions and can't easily talk during them. Active labor typically lasts 4-8 hours for first babies, shorter for subsequent babies.

Transition (8-10 cm dilation): The most intense phase. Contractions are very strong, very close together (2-3 minutes apart), lasting 60-90 seconds. Many people feel overwhelmed, nauseous, shaky during transition. This phase typically lasts 30 minutes to 2 hours. It's hardest but shortest.

Second stage (pushing and birth): From full dilation (10 cm) until baby is born. For first babies, pushing typically lasts 1-3 hours. For subsequent babies, often under an hour. Some people feel immediate urge to push. Others need coaching to find the urge.

Third stage (placenta delivery): After baby is born, the placenta detaches and is delivered. This typically happens 5-30 minutes after birth. Contractions resume (much milder than labor contractions) to help placenta deliver.

Research shows first-time mothers average 12-18 hours of labor from active labor onset to birth, while subsequent labors average 6-8 hours, though tremendous variation exists (Albers, 1999).

18.2 Early Labor at Home

Most people spend early labor at home because going to the hospital too early often leads to unnecessary interventions. Unless complications arise, staying home during early labor is optimal.

What early labor feels like:

- Irregular or regular contractions that gradually intensify
- Cramping similar to menstrual cramps
- Lower back ache
- Possible bloody show (mucus plug discharge tinged with blood)

- Possible water breaking (though this happens before labor for only about 10% of people)
- Excitement mixed with nervousness
- Possible burst of energy (nesting urge intensifies)

Coping strategies for early labor:

Rest if it's night: If labor starts at night and contractions are mild, sleep between contractions. You'll need energy later. This is easier said than done with adrenaline and excitement, but rest when possible.

Stay active if it's day: If labor starts during waking hours and you feel energetic, stay gently active. Walk, do light household tasks, stay upright. Movement helps labor progress.

Eat and drink: Eat light, easily digestible foods. Stay hydrated. Once you're in active labor, you might not want food, and hospital policies sometimes restrict eating during labor.

Distraction: Watch movies, play games, take a bath (warm water often helps with early contractions). Don't obsess over timing every contraction yet.

When to start timing contractions: Once contractions become regular and require your focused attention, start timing them. Track how far apart they are (from start of one to start of next) and how long each lasts. Several apps make this easy.

When to call your provider: Follow the guidelines your provider gave you, typically:

- Regular contractions 5 minutes apart, lasting 1 minute each, for 1 hour (the "5-1-1 rule") for first babies
- Sooner for subsequent babies (often 10-1-1 or even earlier since labor progresses faster)
- Immediately if water breaks, if bleeding heavily, if baby's movement decreases significantly, or if you have severe pain

18.3 Active Labor Coping

Active labor is intense. Contractions demand your complete focus. Coping techniques help you manage pain and work with your body.

Movement and positioning:

Stay upright and mobile when possible: Walking, swaying, slow dancing with your partner, standing and leaning on support—upright positions use gravity to help baby descend and often reduce pain compared to lying down.

Try various positions: Hands and knees, squatting (supported or using birth stool), sitting on birth ball, side-lying, standing and leaning forward. Different positions feel better at different times. Change positions frequently.

Avoid flat on back: Lying flat on your back compresses major blood vessels and can reduce blood flow to baby. It also fights gravity. If you need to lie down, lie on your side.

Breathing techniques:

Slow, deep breathing: Breathe slowly and deeply during contractions. This provides oxygen, prevents hyperventilation, and gives you something to focus on. Count breaths if that helps—breathe in for 4 counts, out for 6 counts.

Vocalization: Low, deep moaning or humming during contractions helps some people. Low sounds relax your pelvic floor. High-pitched sounds tense it. If you're vocalizing, keep sounds low and deep.

Don't hold your breath: Keep breathing throughout contractions. Holding your breath increases pain and reduces oxygen to you and baby.

Physical comfort measures:

Water: Shower or bath (if water hasn't broken) often provides significant relief. Warm water relaxes muscles and reduces pain perception. Some people labor entirely in water.

Counterpressure: Firm pressure on your lower back during contractions can relieve back pain. Partners provide counterpressure with hands, fists, or massage tools.

Massage: Light touch massage, firm pressure, whatever feels good. Some people find touch overwhelming during intense labor—tell your support people what you need.

Heat or cold: Heating pad, warm compresses, ice packs—use whatever provides relief.

Mental coping:

Stay present: Focus on one contraction at a time. Don't think about hours ahead. Just this contraction, right now.

Visualization: Imagine your cervix opening, baby descending, contractions doing productive work. Some people visualize waves, flowers opening, or other imagery.

Mantras: Short phrases you repeat: "I can do this." "My body knows how to birth." "One contraction closer." Whatever resonates with you.

Remember it's finite: Labor has an endpoint. This intensity is temporary. You will get through it.

18.4 Transition

Transition—the final phase of first stage labor, from 8-10 cm dilation—is the most intense part of labor. Many people describe it as the hardest but also the shortest phase.

What transition feels like:

- Overwhelming intensity
- Contractions very close together with little rest between
- Nausea or vomiting
- Shaking, trembling
- Feeling like you can't continue
- Emotional intensity—fear, doubt, wanting to quit
- Often announcing "I can't do this anymore"

The paradox: When you feel like you can't continue, you're almost done. Transition typically lasts 30 minutes to 2 hours. It's the hardest part, but it means you're close to pushing and birth.

Coping with transition:

Support from others: Transition is when you most need support people to remind you that you can do this, that this is normal, that you're almost done.

One contraction at a time: Transition is so intense that you literally can only focus on the immediate moment. Let support people worry about the big picture. You focus on right now.

Vocalization: Many people vocalize intensely during transition. Low sounds, moaning, roaring—whatever helps.

Position changes: Sometimes changing positions provides brief relief or helps labor progress.

Remember this is temporary: Transition is finite. You're about to meet your baby.

18.5 Pushing and Birth

Once you're fully dilated to 10 cm, you enter second stage—pushing and birth. For many people, pushing feels like relief after transition because you can actively do something rather than just enduring contractions.

What pushing feels like:

Many people feel overwhelming urge to push—your body involuntarily pushes. Some describe it as needing to have the largest bowel movement ever. Others don't feel clear urge and need coaching to find the pushing sensation.

Types of pushing:

Spontaneous pushing: Following your body's urge to push. When you feel the urge, you push. Between urges, you rest. This is physiologic pushing and often works well.

Directed pushing: Provider or nurse coaching you when to push and how long. "Take a deep breath, hold it, push for 10 counts." This is sometimes necessary but not always optimal.

Research suggests spontaneous pushing with breath-holding under 6 seconds reduces perineal damage compared to directed pushing with long breath-holds (Prins et al., 2011).

Pushing positions:

You can push in many positions—not just flat on your back with legs in stirrups (though that's traditional medical model). Options include:

- Side-lying
- Semi-sitting
- Squatting (supported or using squat bar)
- Hands and knees
- Standing
- Birth stool

Upright positions use gravity and increase pelvic opening, potentially making pushing more effective.

The ring of fire: As baby's head crowns (emerges through vaginal opening), intense burning or stinging sensation occurs. This is the "ring of fire" and means birth is imminent. It typically lasts just seconds to a minute.

Birth moment: Baby's head emerges, then body follows quickly (usually within 1-2 contractions). Baby takes first breaths, cries, and is placed on your chest (or your partner's chest if you prefer). The work is done. You've given birth.

18.6 The Midwifery Model

The midwifery model of care differs philosophically from the medical model, emphasizing physiologic birth, minimal intervention, and supporting the birthing person's body to do what it's designed to do.

Midwifery principles:

- Birth is a normal physiologic process, not a medical emergency
- Bodies know how to give birth
- Interventions should be used only when medically indicated, not routinely
- Support and patience often work better than intervention
- Birthing people should be active participants in decisions
- Continuous support during labor improves outcomes

Evidence supports midwifery approach: Studies show that midwifery care results in fewer interventions, fewer cesareans, higher satisfaction, and similar or better outcomes compared to physician care for low-risk pregnancies (Sandall et al., 2016).

What this looks like practically:

- Encouraging movement and position changes
- Using non-pharmacological comfort measures first

- Avoiding routine interventions (continuous monitoring, IV, breaking water, restricting food/drink)
- Patient laboring and pushing rather than physician directing everything
- Respecting the body's timeline rather than rushing labor

LGBTQ+ families and midwifery: Midwifery practices are often more progressive and LGBTQ+-affirming than large hospital systems. Many LGBTQ+ families choose midwives specifically for more personalized, respectful care.

18.7 Partner Support Throughout Labor

Partners play crucial roles supporting the laboring person physically, emotionally, and practically.

Physical support:

- Provide counterpressure on lower back during contractions
- Hold them during contractions (supporting while standing, holding hands while squatting)
- Help with position changes
- Offer water, ice chips, cool washcloth
- Massage back, feet, hands, or wherever feels good
- Apply heat or cold packs

Emotional support:

- Remind them they can do this
- Provide reassurance during intense moments
- Tell them they're doing great
- Remind them labor is finite—they're getting closer
- Stay calm even when they're overwhelmed
- Be present without needing to fix everything

Practical support:

- Track contractions so laboring person doesn't have to

- Communicate with medical staff
- Make sure birth preferences are followed
- Be the bad guy if necessary ("She said she doesn't want an epidural offered unless she asks")
- Protect laboring person's space and energy

What not to do:

- Don't take it personally if they snap at you or say they hate you during transition
- Don't be offended if they don't want to be touched
- Don't tell them to be quiet if they're vocalizing
- Don't leave the room except briefly unless they say it's okay
- Don't panic—stay calm even when labor is intense

For LGBTQ+ partners specifically: You're also becoming a parent today. This is your baby's birth too. Be present, involved, and take it seriously. But also know your primary role during labor is supporting your partner—your active parenting starts once baby arrives.

18.8 Pain Management Options

Pain management during labor exists on a spectrum from no medication to complete pain relief via epidural.

Non-pharmacological options:

- Movement and positioning
- Water (shower, bath, birth tub)
- Breathing and vocalization
- Massage and counterpressure
- Heat and cold
- Hypnosis or visualization
- TENS unit (electrical nerve stimulation)
- Aromatherapy
- Music

Nitrous oxide (where available): Inhaled gas that reduces pain perception without eliminating sensation. Benefits include staying mobile and alert, you control when you use it, no major side effects. Limitations include it only dulls pain rather than eliminating it, and some people find it causes nausea.

IV pain medications: Opioids given through IV provide pain relief without the restrictions of epidural. Benefits include pain reduction while maintaining some mobility. Limitations include drowsiness, nausea, medications cross placenta potentially affecting baby, and pain relief is less complete than epidural.

Epidural analgesia: Medication delivered through catheter into epidural space of spine that numbs lower body. Benefits include very effective pain relief, ability to rest during long labor. Limitations include restricted mobility (in bed once placed), potential to slow labor, increased chance of interventions, rare but possible complications, and interventions cascade (epidural often requires continuous monitoring, IV fluids, urinary catheter).

Making decisions: No decision is permanent. You can plan unmedicated birth and change your mind. You can plan epidural and find you don't need it. You can try other methods first and get epidural later if pain becomes overwhelming. There's no award for suffering. There's also no shame in unmedicated birth if that's what you want. Your labor, your choice.

18.9 Real Labor Story

Consider Maria and Sofia's birth experience (composite): Maria's labor started at 2am with mild contractions. She labored at home until noon, when contractions were five minutes apart and intense enough that she couldn't talk through them. They went to the hospital.

Maria was 5 centimeters dilated. She walked the halls, swayed with Sofia supporting her, labored in the shower. By 4pm, she was 7 centimeters and contractions were overwhelming. She asked for pain relief.

She initially tried IV medication, but it only dulled the pain and made her drowsy without providing real relief. At 6pm, now 8 centimeters, she requested an epidural. The anesthesiologist placed it, and within 20 minutes, Maria felt significant relief.

She rested for an hour, dilating to 10 centimeters during that time. At 8pm, she started pushing. The epidural had worn down enough that she could feel pressure and work with contractions. Sofia held one leg while a nurse held the other. After 90 minutes of pushing, their son was born at 9:30pm.

Maria had wanted unmedicated birth but changed her mind in the moment—and felt good about that decision. The epidural let her rest and arrive at pushing with energy rather than exhausted. Both mothers held their son immediately, crying and laughing. Labor hadn't gone exactly as planned, but their baby was here and they'd done it together.

18.10 Core Labor Principles

Labor progresses through distinct stages: early labor (typically spent at home), active labor (intense regular contractions), transition (most intense phase from 8-10 cm), pushing, and placenta delivery. Each phase requires different coping strategies.

Early labor benefits from rest, light activity, and distraction. Active labor requires focused coping—movement, positioning, breathing, physical comfort measures, and mental strategies. Transition is the hardest but shortest phase, requiring intensive support and one-contraction-at-a-time focus. Pushing often feels like relief because you can actively participate.

The midwifery model emphasizes physiologic birth, minimal intervention, and supporting the body's natural process. Partners provide crucial physical, emotional, and practical support throughout. Pain management exists on a spectrum from unmedicated to epidural, and changing your mind during labor is completely acceptable.

Labor is intense, unpredictable, and deeply transformative. Understanding what to expect, having coping tools, and surrounding yourself with good support creates the best possible foundation for birth.

Chapter 19.0: Medical Interventions and Cesareans

Isabella's labor was going well until it wasn't. After 18 hours, progress stalled at 9 centimeters. The baby's heart rate started showing decelerations during contractions. Isabella was exhausted. The obstetrician recommended a cesarean. Carmen held Isabella's hand while they both cried—this wasn't the birth they'd planned—and then agreed. Their daughter was born 30 minutes later via cesarean, healthy and perfect. The birth didn't match their plan, but their baby was safe.

Labor doesn't always progress smoothly. Medical interventions—induction, epidural, continuous monitoring, assisted delivery, cesarean birth—are sometimes necessary to ensure safety for the birthing person and baby. Understanding when and why interventions are recommended helps you make informed decisions. This chapter covers common interventions, cesarean birth (planned and emergency), gentle cesarean techniques, and recovery.

19.1 When Interventions Become Necessary

The goal is physiologic birth with minimal intervention when possible, but interventions exist because sometimes they save lives or prevent serious complications.

Legitimate reasons for interventions:

- Labor not progressing after adequate time
- Baby showing signs of distress
- Birthing person's health at risk (severe hypertension, bleeding, exhaustion)
- Placental problems (abruption, previa)

- Cord prolapse (umbilical cord comes through cervix before baby)
- Baby in distress position (persistent transverse or breech position)
- Hemorrhage
- Infection

Interventions cascade: One intervention often leads to others. For example, epidural might slow labor, leading to Pitocin augmentation, leading to stronger contractions, leading to fetal heart rate changes, leading to cesarean. This doesn't mean epidurals are bad—just that interventions have downstream effects to consider.

Questions to ask when intervention is suggested:

- Why is this being recommended?
- What happens if we wait/don't do this?
- What are the benefits and risks?
- Are there alternatives?
- Can we have time to discuss this privately? (unless it's an emergency)

Trust your providers, but advocate: Good providers recommend interventions for legitimate reasons. But you're allowed to ask questions, understand reasoning, and participate in decisions. True emergencies requiring immediate action are rare. Most situations allow time for discussion.

19.2 Induction of Labor

Induction means starting labor artificially before it begins spontaneously. About 25% of pregnancies involve induction (Martin et al., 2021).

Medical reasons for induction:

- Pregnancy beyond 41-42 weeks (post-dates)

- Water broke but labor hasn't started (and it's been 12-24+ hours)
- Medical conditions (hypertension, diabetes, cholestasis)
- Placental problems
- Decreased amniotic fluid
- Baby's growth problems
- Concerns about baby's wellbeing

Non-medical induction: Some inductions happen for logistical reasons (provider going out of town, birthing person wanting to schedule birth). Elective induction before 39 weeks is generally not recommended. After 39 weeks, recent research suggests induction might reduce cesarean rates compared to expectant management, though this is debated (Grobman et al., 2018).

Induction methods:

Cervical ripening (if cervix isn't favorable): Medications (prostaglandins like misoprostol or dinoprostone) or mechanical methods (Foley balloon catheter) to soften and dilate cervix before active labor induction begins.

Breaking water (artificial rupture of membranes): If cervix is favorable, breaking the bag of waters often starts or strengthens contractions.

Pitocin (synthetic oxytocin): IV medication that causes contractions. Dose is gradually increased until contractions are regular and strong.

Induction challenges: Induced labor is often more painful than spontaneous labor because Pitocin creates stronger, closer contractions. Induction success varies—some people deliver within hours, others take days of induction before labor establishes or before deciding on cesarean.

For LGBTQ+ families: Induction doesn't change the fact that both parents are equally important. Make sure providers include both parents in induction discussions and decisions.

19.3 Epidural Analgesia

Epidurals are the most effective labor pain management option, providing significant to complete pain relief for most people.

How epidurals work: Anesthesiologist inserts a catheter into the epidural space surrounding the spinal cord. Medication is delivered continuously through this catheter, numbing nerves from belly down to legs.

Placement process: You sit or lie on your side in a curved position. The anesthesiologist cleans your back, gives local anesthetic to numb the skin, then inserts the epidural catheter. Once placed, medication is delivered continuously. Most people feel relief within 15-20 minutes.

Benefits:

- Significant pain relief (most people report 80-100% pain reduction)
- Ability to rest during long labor
- If cesarean becomes necessary, epidural can be increased for surgery without needing general anesthesia

Limitations and side effects:

- Restricted to bed once placed (can't walk with epidural)
- Blood pressure drop (treated with IV fluids)
- Might slow labor (sometimes requiring Pitocin augmentation)
- Increased need for urinary catheter, continuous monitoring
- Possible "hot spots" where pain relief is incomplete
- Rare complications (spinal headache, nerve damage—both very rare)
- Might make pushing harder since you can't feel contractions as clearly

Epidurals don't:

- Cause permanent back pain (myth—research shows no long-term back problems from epidural)
- Paralyze you (extremely rare complication, not typical effect)
- Harm baby directly (medication stays in epidural space, very little crosses to baby)

Decision-making: Epidural is neither mandatory nor forbidden. It's a tool. If pain is overwhelming and preventing you from coping with labor, epidural might help. If you're managing without it, you don't need it. Both approaches are valid.

19.4 Continuous Monitoring

Continuous electronic fetal monitoring tracks baby's heart rate and uterine contractions throughout labor via monitors on your belly or internal monitors (after water breaks).

Why it's done: Monitors detect concerning heart rate patterns that might indicate baby is stressed or not getting enough oxygen.

Benefits: Identifies babies in distress who need intervention.

Limitations:

- Restricts movement (tethered to monitors)
- High false positive rate (monitors show concerning patterns that aren't actually problems, leading to unnecessary interventions)
- Doesn't improve outcomes for low-risk pregnancies compared to intermittent monitoring

Research shows: For low-risk pregnancies, intermittent monitoring (checking heart rate every 15-30 minutes with handheld device) works as well as continuous monitoring with fewer interventions (Alfirevic et al., 2017). For high-risk pregnancies, continuous monitoring provides important information.

Alternatives: Request intermittent monitoring if you're low-risk. This allows movement and positioning changes while still tracking baby's wellbeing.

19.5 Assisted Delivery

Vacuum extraction or forceps-assisted delivery helps guide baby out during pushing when baby is low in birth canal but not descending adequately.

Vacuum: Suction device attached to baby's head that provider uses to help guide baby out while you push.

Forceps: Metal instruments resembling large salad tongs that cradle baby's head, helping provider guide baby out during contractions.

When they're used:

- Prolonged pushing without progress (baby is close but not quite delivering)
- Baby showing signs of distress during pushing
- Birthing person exhausted and can't push effectively
- Medical conditions making prolonged pushing dangerous

Risks: Possible bruising or temporary marks on baby's head (usually resolve quickly), small increased risk of perineal tearing for birthing person.

Alternative: Cesarean birth if assisted delivery fails or isn't appropriate.

19.6 Cesarean Birth Overview

Cesarean birth (C-section) is surgical delivery through incisions in abdomen and uterus. About 32% of U.S. births are cesarean (Martin et al., 2021).

Planned (scheduled) cesarean reasons:

- Baby in breech or transverse position
- Placenta previa (placenta covering cervix)
- Previous uterine surgery or cesarean (though VBAC—vaginal birth after cesarean—is often possible)
- Twins or higher-order multiples (depending on positions)
- Certain maternal health conditions
- Baby's size concerns (though this is controversial)

Emergency cesarean reasons:

- Labor not progressing after adequate time
- Baby showing signs of severe distress
- Umbilical cord prolapse
- Placental abruption
- Hemorrhage
- Other complications requiring immediate delivery

Urgent versus true emergency: Most "emergency" cesareans are actually "urgent"—they need to happen soon (within 30-60 minutes) but not within minutes. True stat emergencies requiring immediate surgery are rare.

19.7 Cesarean Procedure

Understanding what happens during cesarean helps reduce fear.

Preparation:

- Epidural is increased for surgery, or spinal anesthesia is placed (provides numbness from chest down)
- Catheter is placed to drain bladder
- Belly is cleaned and draped
- Partner wears scrubs and sits by your head (usually behind a screen so you don't see the surgery)

Surgery:

- Incision is made in lower abdomen (typically horizontal "bikini cut")
- Layers of tissue are separated to reach uterus
- Incision is made in uterus
- Baby is lifted out (you might feel pressure and pulling but not pain)
- Umbilical cord is clamped and cut
- Baby is briefly evaluated by pediatric team
- Baby is usually brought to you for skin-to-skin (or to partner if you're not able)
- Placenta is removed
- Uterus and abdominal layers are sutured closed

Duration: Surgery typically takes 45-60 minutes total, though baby is born within first 5-10 minutes. Most of the time involves suturing layers closed.

19.8 Gentle Cesarean Techniques

Gentle (family-centered) cesarean incorporates elements that make the experience more positive while maintaining safety.

Gentle cesarean options:

- Clear drape or drape lowered so you can watch baby being born
- Arms free (not strapped down)
- Immediate skin-to-skin in operating room
- Delayed cord clamping if baby is stable
- Partner present throughout
- Both parents able to hold baby in OR
- Music playing
- Dimmed lights
- Narrating what's happening so you feel involved

Ask about gentle cesarean: If cesarean is planned or becomes necessary, ask if your hospital offers gentle cesarean techniques. Many hospitals now incorporate these practices.

For LGBTQ+ families: Make sure both parents can be present, both hold baby, and both are included in what's happening. "My wife is a mother to this baby—she should be able to hold the baby in the OR just like I would."

19.9 Cesarean Recovery

Cesarean recovery is more challenging than vaginal birth recovery because you're healing from major abdominal surgery while caring for a newborn.

Hospital recovery (typically 2-4 days):

- Pain management (usually combination of medications)
- Catheter remains for first 12-24 hours
- Encouraged to walk within 12-24 hours (helps prevent blood clots and speeds recovery)
- Monitoring incision, bleeding, vital signs
- Supporting infant feeding
- Learning to care for baby while managing post-surgical pain

Home recovery (6-8 weeks):

- Incision care (keeping clean and dry, watching for infection signs)
- Pain management
- Avoiding heavy lifting and strenuous activity
- Getting in and out of bed carefully
- Using pillow to support incision when coughing or laughing
- Walking regularly but not overdoing it

Physical limitations: Don't lift anything heavier than baby for at least 2 weeks. Don't drive until you can brake forcefully without pain (usually 1-2 weeks). Don't exercise beyond walking until 6-8 weeks and cleared by provider.

Emotional recovery: Cesarean can bring complicated emotions—relief that baby is safe, grief that vaginal birth didn't happen, feeling like you failed (you didn't—cesarean is birth). Process these feelings with partners, friends, or therapists. VBAC is often possible for future births if you want it.

19.10 Example of Unexpected Cesarean

Consider Priya and Nicole's experience (composite): Priya labored for 22 hours. By hour 18, she was dilated to 9 centimeters and had been there for 4 hours without progressing further. The baby's heart rate started showing late decelerations—drops after contractions ended, a concerning pattern.

The obstetrician recommended cesarean. Priya and Nicole asked questions: Could they wait longer? The OB explained that lack of progress after 4 hours at 9 centimeters combined with heart rate changes suggested the baby wasn't tolerating labor well. Waiting risked the baby's wellbeing.

They agreed to cesarean, both crying. Nicole put on scrubs and stayed with Priya throughout. The surgery team explained everything as it happened. When their daughter was born, the pediatric team quickly checked her, confirmed she was stable, and brought her directly to Priya for skin-to-skin on the operating table.

Nicole held Priya's hand, then got to hold their daughter while Priya was being closed. Both mothers were in tears—their daughter was here, safe, even though the birth looked nothing like they'd planned.

Recovery was hard. Priya needed help getting out of bed, couldn't pick up the baby easily, and felt frustrated by her body's limitations. But within two weeks, she felt significantly better. By six weeks, recovery was complete.

Looking back, they wished they hadn't needed cesarean but recognized it was the right decision for their baby's safety. The birth didn't go as planned, but what mattered was that their daughter was healthy and they were a family.

19.11 Critical Intervention Insights

Medical interventions during labor—induction, epidural, continuous monitoring, assisted delivery, cesarean birth—exist because they're sometimes necessary for safety. Understanding when and why interventions are recommended allows informed participation in decisions.

Induction starts labor artificially for medical reasons or occasionally for logistics. Epidural provides effective pain relief but comes with limitations including restricted mobility. Continuous monitoring tracks baby's wellbeing but restricts movement and has high false positive rates.

Cesarean birth is surgical delivery through abdominal incisions, performed for planned medical reasons or urgently when complications arise. Gentle cesarean techniques make the experience more positive. Cesarean recovery takes 6-8 weeks and involves healing from major surgery while caring for a newborn.

Not all births follow the ideal plan. Interventions and cesarean don't mean failure—they're tools that sometimes save lives. The measure of a good birth isn't whether it matches your plan, but whether everyone is healthy and you feel respected throughout.

Chapter 20.0: Trans Birth Considerations

Marcus went into labor at 39 weeks. His husband Tao drove him to the hospital where staff had been prepped about his case—transgender man giving birth, use he/him pronouns, refer to chest not breasts, both parents are fathers. Most of the labor staff were respectful. But during pushing, a new nurse came on shift who hadn't been briefed. She kept saying "Good job, mama" until Marcus, in the middle of a contraction, shouted "I'm not a fucking mother, I'm a father!" Tao immediately advocated, the nurse apologized and corrected, but the damage was done. Marcus felt dysphoric and violated during the most vulnerable moment of his life.

Birth for transgender and non-binary people involves unique challenges: managing chest exposure, handling pelvic exams during labor, dealing with gendered language when you're physically vulnerable, educating staff in the moment, managing dysphoria during intense physical experience, and ensuring partners can advocate effectively. This chapter addresses birth-specific considerations for trans and non-binary pregnant people, covering dysphoria management during labor, staff education, trauma-informed care, and advocacy strategies.

20.1 Managing Chest Exposure

Labor and birth often involve being partially or fully undressed. For transgender men and non-binary people, particularly those who haven't had top surgery, chest exposure can trigger severe dysphoria.

Why exposure happens:

- Skin-to-skin contact immediately after birth (baby placed on bare chest)
- Monitoring heart rate and contractions (monitors on belly, sometimes chest)
- Physical exams
- Assistance with chest-feeding if applicable

Strategies for managing:

Communicate preferences clearly: In your birth plan and verbally when you arrive, state: "I experience dysphoria with chest exposure. Please minimize this as much as medically possible."

Stay clothed longer: Wear a hospital gown or your own clothing as long as possible during labor. You don't need to be naked for most of labor.

Strategic exposure: If skin-to-skin is important to you but chest exposure is triggering, consider brief skin-to-skin immediately after birth (with baby covering most of your chest) then quickly wrap yourself or transfer baby to partner.

Partner skin-to-skin first: Some trans men prefer their partner to do first skin-to-skin so they can avoid chest exposure entirely. "My partner will do skin-to-skin first. I'll hold the baby while clothed or wrapped."

Sports bra or binder (carefully): Some transgender men wear sports bras during labor for coverage. Binding during labor is generally not recommended (restricts breathing when you need maximum oxygen), but a loose sports bra provides coverage without tight compression.

Draping: Request towels or blankets for coverage whenever you're not actively being examined.

If you've had top surgery: Chest exposure might be less triggering post-surgery, though you might still want coverage for comfort or privacy. Communicate your preferences.

20.2 Pelvic Exams During Labor

Labor involves multiple pelvic exams to check cervical dilation, baby's position, and progress. For many transgender men and non-binary people, pelvic exams during labor trigger intense dysphoria.

When pelvic exams happen:

- Initial assessment when you arrive at hospital (checking current dilation)
- Periodically during labor to assess progress (every 2-4 hours typically)
- Before pushing to confirm full dilation
- After birth to check for tears and repair if necessary

Minimizing dysphoria during exams:

Communicate with providers: "Pelvic exams trigger dysphoria. Please do only medically necessary exams, explain what you're doing, and check in with me."

Use preferred language: "Please use the terms 'front hole' [or whatever term you prefer] rather than vagina." Providers should use your language during exams.

Bring support: Have your partner present during exams, holding your hand, talking to you, providing distraction.

Distraction techniques: Focus on breathing, listen to music with headphones, count ceiling tiles, talk with partner about something unrelated.

Limit number of examiners: Request that the same provider do all pelvic exams rather than multiple different people examining you. This reduces repeated violations of your space.

Verbal narration: Ask providers to tell you what they're doing before and during exams. Knowing what to expect reduces trauma.

Remember purpose: These exams serve medical purposes—monitoring your labor progress and ensuring safety. They're temporary and purposeful, even though they trigger dysphoria.

20.3 Gendered Language During Birth

Labor is often when gendered language becomes most intense and most painful for trans and non-binary people. You're physically vulnerable, in pain, unable to advocate for yourself effectively, and people keep calling you "mom" or "mama" despite corrections.

Common language problems:

- Nurses saying "Good job, mama!" during contractions
- Providers referring to "mother and baby"
- Instructions like "Push like you're having a bowel movement, mommy!"
- Paperwork and wristbands saying "mother"
- Assumptions about chest-feeding ("Let's get mama nursing!")

Preventing language problems:

Chart notes: Ensure your chart has prominent notes about pronouns and language. Patient advocates should have added these weeks before you went into labor (see Chapter 17.0).

Birth plan: First page of birth plan should state pronouns and preferred language in large, bold text.

Verbal reminder on arrival: When you arrive in labor, state immediately: "I'm Marcus, I use he/him pronouns, I'm the father not the mother. Please make sure everyone knows this."

Shift changes: Each time nursing staff changes shifts, your partner should remind new staff about pronouns and language. "Just so you know, he uses he/him pronouns and is the father. Please use masculine language."

Partners as language police: Your partner's job includes correcting language mistakes so you don't have to during contractions. When a nurse says "mama," your partner immediately says "He's the father, not mother—please use 'he' and 'dad.'"

20.4 Staff Education in the Moment

Despite advance preparation, many labor and delivery staff will have little to no experience with transgender pregnancy. Some education happens in real time during your labor.

What's reasonable to expect:

Basic respect: Staff should use your stated pronouns and name consistently after being told once. Occasional mistakes happen under stress, but they should correct immediately when reminded.

Willingness to learn: Staff don't need to fully understand transgender pregnancy, but they should be willing to use your language and follow your lead.

Asking questions appropriately: Questions for understanding your needs are fine. Invasive personal questions about your body, transition, or sex life are not appropriate.

What's not acceptable:

Refusing to use pronouns: If staff actively refuse or dismissively ignore your pronouns, that's discrimination. Escalate to charge nurse or patient advocate immediately.

Making it about them: Staff acting shocked, uncomfortable, or treating your pregnancy as entertainment rather than normal medical care is unacceptable.

Requiring you to educate during labor: Basic information is reasonable. Extensive education about transgender issues while you're in active labor is inappropriate—you're busy having a baby.

Realistic expectations: Even in ideal scenarios, you might do some educating. Try to accept that labor staff are learning while providing your care, as frustrating as that is. Focus on whether they're trying and respectful versus demanding perfect understanding immediately.

20.5 Dysphoria During Intense Experience

Labor is the most physically intense experience most people ever have. For transgender men and non-binary people, this intensity combined with dysphoria about body and gendered treatment creates unique challenges.

Why labor intensifies dysphoria:

- Physical vulnerability and lack of control
- Body doing intensely feminine-coded activities (contractions, pushing, giving birth)
- Medical staff touching and examining intimate areas
- Being treated as female despite male identity
- Chest exposure and attention to anatomy
- Feeling trapped in a body doing things you'd rather it wasn't

Coping strategies:

Reframe the experience: Some transgender men find it helpful to view birth as an intensely masculine experience—men's bodies with uteruses doing something powerful and strong. Others mentally separate "what my body is doing" from "who I am." Find the framework that helps you.

Focus on baby: Keep attention on the outcome—meeting your baby—rather than the process of getting there. This is temporary and purposeful.

Partner presence: Having your partner there as a witness to your identity, holding your hand, calling you by your correct name and pronouns, reminds you that you're still you even during this bizarre experience.

Disconnect if necessary: Some people mentally dissociate during labor as a protective mechanism. If this helps you cope, that's okay. You can reconnect with your body and experience later.

Therapy processing: Plan to process the birth experience with a therapist afterward. Labor might be traumatic for trans and non-binary people in ways it isn't for cisgender people. That trauma is valid and deserves support.

20.6 Partner Advocacy

Partners of transgender and non-binary birthing people have critical roles as advocates during labor—protecting their partner from misgendering and discrimination when they're physically unable to advocate for themselves.

What partners should do:

Be the language police: Immediately correct every pronoun mistake, every time. "He, not she." "Father, not mother." Don't let mistakes slide because staff are busy or you don't want to be annoying. Your partner's dignity matters more than staff comfort.

Run interference: If staff are problematic, be the bad guy. Request different nurses, call patient advocates, escalate to supervisors. Protect your partner so they can focus on labor.

Remind staff about language: At every shift change, with every new provider, state: "My partner uses he/him pronouns and is the father. Please use masculine language."

Physical presence: Don't leave the room except briefly. Your presence reminds staff that this is a real person with an identity that matters, not just a fascinating medical case.

After-birth advocacy: If your partner is too dysphoric or exhausted to hold the baby immediately, you hold the baby, do skin-to-skin, and step into active parenting right away. Don't wait for your partner to recover before you engage with your child.

Post-birth support: After birth, continue advocating with postpartum staff about language and respect. The vulnerability doesn't end when labor ends.

20.7 Trauma-Informed Care

Transgender and non-binary people often have trauma histories related to medical systems, discrimination, and body dysphoria. Birth can be retraumatizing without trauma-informed approaches.

Principles of trauma-informed care:

Safety: Creating physical and emotional safety—using correct language, minimizing unnecessary exposure, respecting boundaries.

Trustworthiness and transparency: Explaining what's happening during exams and procedures, asking permission before touching.

Peer support: Connecting with other trans people who've given birth helps normalize the experience.

Collaboration: Including you in decisions rather than doing things to you.

Empowerment: Recognizing your strengths and resilience in navigating pregnancy and birth as trans person.

What trauma-informed providers do:

- Ask permission before touching or examining
- Narrate what they're doing
- Use your language and pronouns consistently
- Validate that this experience is hard
- Check in about how you're coping
- Respect your boundaries
- Recognize past trauma might affect labor experience

Requesting trauma-informed care: "I have trauma history related to medical care and body dysphoria. Can you please ask permission before touching me, explain what you're doing, and check in regularly about how I'm doing?"

20.8 Real Trans Birth Experience

Consider Ravi's birth (composite): Ravi went into labor at midnight. His husband drove him to the hospital where they'd prepped staff about his case. The intake nurse used correct pronouns immediately.

Labor progressed quickly. By 6am, Ravi was in active labor, contractions intense and overwhelming. A new nurse came on shift—she'd been briefed but kept slipping, saying "mama" and "she." Ravi's husband corrected every time. After the fourth correction, the nurse started getting it right.

By noon, Ravi was pushing. The midwife was excellent—using "he" consistently, narrating what she was doing, checking in about dysphoria. When she needed to check for tears after delivery, she asked: "I need to examine you to check for tearing. Is that okay? I'll tell you what I'm seeing."

Ravi's son was born at 1:15pm. The midwife immediately placed him on Ravi's chest. Ravi felt intense conflicting emotions—euphoria at meeting his son, dysphoria at the chest-to-chest contact, pride that his male body had just done this amazing thing, and violation from the exposing, vulnerable experience.

After two minutes of skin-to-skin, Ravi asked his husband to take the baby. His husband did immediate skin-to-skin while Ravi got covered and composed himself. Within ten minutes, Ravi was ready to hold his son again—this time clothed, on his terms.

Recovery was physically hard and emotionally complicated. Ravi processed the birth with his therapist, working through the dysphoria and trauma while celebrating that he'd become a father. Three months postpartum, he resumed testosterone and started feeling like himself again. His son was worth everything.

20.9 Essential Trans Birth Points

Birth for transgender and non-binary people involves managing chest exposure, handling pelvic exams, dealing with gendered language during physical vulnerability, educating staff in the moment, and coping with dysphoria during intensely physical experience. Advance preparation through patient advocates and clear birth plans helps, but real-time advocacy remains necessary.

Partners play crucial roles correcting language, running interference with problematic staff, and protecting their trans partner's dignity when they can't advocate for themselves. Trauma-informed care recognizes past trauma and current dysphoria, prioritizing safety, transparency, and empowerment.

Labor can be traumatic for trans and non-binary people in unique ways. This trauma deserves validation and processing with supportive therapists. Birth as a trans or non-binary person requires enormous strength and resilience. You can do hard things, and becoming a parent is worth the difficult journey.

Part Five: Postpartum And Feeding

Chapter 21.0: Immediate Postpartum Hours

Isabella held her daughter for the first time at 11:47pm. The baby was warm, wet, screaming, and absolutely perfect. Carmen cut the umbilical cord with shaking hands while crying. The midwife placed the baby on Isabella's chest, skin-to-skin, and covered them both with warm blankets. Time stopped. Nothing existed except this tiny human they'd created, finally here, finally real.

The first hours after birth are intense and magical—a blur of emotions, physical sensations, medical procedures, and meeting your baby. For LGBTQ+ families, these hours also involve ensuring both parents bond with baby, establishing feeding plans, and making decisions about newborn care. This chapter covers skin-to-skin contact, placenta delivery, perineal repair, newborn procedures, partner bonding, first feeding attempts, and going home.

21.1 Skin to Skin Contact

Immediate skin-to-skin contact—placing baby directly on the birthing person's bare chest right after birth—provides significant benefits for both baby and parents.

Benefits of skin-to-skin:

- Regulates baby's temperature, heart rate, and breathing
- Stabilizes blood sugar
- Reduces baby's stress hormones
- Promotes bonding and attachment
- Facilitates early breastfeeding or chest-feeding
- Releases oxytocin in birthing person, helping uterus contract and reducing bleeding

Research shows that babies who have immediate skin-to-skin contact cry less, maintain better body temperature, and are more likely to successfully initiate feeding compared to babies who are separated from parents after birth (Moore et al., 2016).

How skin-to-skin works: Immediately after birth, before weighing, measuring, or bathing, the baby is placed on the birthing person's bare chest. A blanket covers both of them. Baby stays there for at least the first hour, often longer.

For LGBTQ+ families: Both parents should get skin-to-skin time in the first hours. Typically, the gestational parent has first contact immediately after birth. After 30-60 minutes, the non-gestational partner can have skin-to-skin time while the gestational parent rests, gets stitches if needed, or showers.

For transgender men and non-binary people: Skin-to-skin might trigger dysphoria due to chest exposure. You can modify this: brief skin-to-skin immediately after birth (with baby covering most of your chest), then transfer baby to partner for extended skin-to-skin. Or skip it entirely and have your partner do immediate skin-to-skin. Both options support bonding—do what feels bearable for you.

21.2 Placenta Delivery

After baby is born, you're not quite done—the placenta still needs to deliver. This is the third stage of labor.

What happens: Within 5-30 minutes after baby's birth, the placenta detaches from the uterine wall. You'll feel contractions (much milder than labor contractions) and might be asked to push gently. The placenta slides out, followed by the umbilical cord.

Active management versus physiologic: Most providers use active management—giving you medication (typically Pitocin) after birth to help the uterus contract and reduce bleeding. Physiologic management means waiting for the placenta to deliver naturally without medication. Active management reduces risk of postpartum hemorrhage slightly (Begley et al., 2019).

Delayed cord clamping: Many providers now wait 1-3 minutes after birth before clamping and cutting the umbilical cord, allowing more blood to transfer from placenta to baby. This improves baby's iron stores and may have other health benefits.

What it feels like: Placenta delivery is anticlimactic after giving birth to a baby. It's squishy, wet, and over quickly. Most people barely notice it because they're focused on their baby.

21.3 Perineal Repair

If vaginal tearing occurred during birth (common for first-time births), the provider will examine and repair tears after placenta delivery.

Degrees of tearing:

- First degree: Superficial skin tears, often heal without stitches
- Second degree: Deeper tears into muscle, require stitches
- Third and fourth degree: Severe tears extending into anal sphincter (less common)

Repair process: If you had epidural, it's still working and you won't feel repair. If you didn't have epidural, the provider uses local anesthetic to numb the area before stitching. Repair typically takes 15-30 minutes.

For transgender men: Perineal examination and repair can trigger severe dysphoria. Having your partner present, using distraction techniques, and communicating with your provider helps. Remember this is temporary medical care that's necessary for healing.

After repair: Stitches are dissolvable and don't need to be removed. The area will be sore for 1-2 weeks. Ice packs, witch hazel pads, and pain medication help. Most people feel significantly better by two weeks postpartum.

21.4 Newborn Procedures

Several routine procedures happen in the first hours after birth. You consent or decline for each.

Immediate procedures (first minutes):

- Drying baby and assessing breathing
- Assigning Apgar scores at 1 minute and 5 minutes (measures baby's color, heart rate, reflexes, muscle tone, breathing)
- Cutting umbilical cord (after delayed clamping if you requested it)

Within first hour:

- Weighing and measuring (can be delayed until after first hour of skin-to-skin)
- Vitamin K injection (prevents bleeding disorders—strongly recommended)
- Erythromycin eye ointment (prevents eye infections from bacteria encountered during birth—many parents consent but some decline if STI screening was negative)
- Identification bands placed on baby's ankle and parents' wrists

Within 24 hours:

- Hepatitis B vaccine (first dose)
- Hearing screening
- Newborn metabolic screening (heel stick blood test that screens for genetic and metabolic disorders)
- Pulse oximetry screening (checks oxygen levels to detect heart defects)

- Physical exam by pediatrician

Decision-making: Discuss which procedures you consent to and which you decline. Most medical organizations strongly recommend vitamin K injection and metabolic screening. Other procedures involve more individual decision-making.

21.5 Partner Holding and Bonding

Non-gestational partners often feel left out immediately after birth because the gestational parent is holding the baby. Intentional partner bonding time matters.

When partner should hold baby: After the gestational parent has had 30-60 minutes of initial skin-to-skin and bonding, the non-gestational partner should have extended holding and skin-to-skin time.

Skin-to-skin for partners: Non-gestational partners can and should do skin-to-skin. Remove your shirt, hold baby on your bare chest, cover both of you with a blanket. This provides the same regulation and bonding benefits as skin-to-skin with the gestational parent.

Why this matters: Research shows that non-gestational parents who have early skin-to-skin contact and holding time report stronger attachment to babies and better co-parenting relationships (Shorey et al., 2016). Don't wait days to hold your baby—engage immediately.

For lesbian couples: Both mothers should have equal access to baby from the start. Make sure medical staff recognize that the non-gestational mother is also a parent, not just a support person.

For partners of transgender men: You might do first skin-to-skin if your partner is too dysphoric for chest exposure. This isn't a lesser option—it's protecting your partner's mental health while ensuring baby gets skin-to-skin benefits.

21.6 First Feeding Attempt

Most babies are alert and interested in feeding within the first hour after birth. This is an optimal time for first feeding attempt if you're chest-feeding or breastfeeding.

If chest-feeding or breastfeeding: With baby on your chest during skin-to-skin, baby will often naturally move toward the breast or chest and attempt to latch. This is called the "breast crawl." Midwives or nurses can help with positioning and latch.

First attempts are often clumsy. Baby might lick, nuzzle, or just rest near the nipple before latching. That's normal. The first feeding might last 5 minutes or 30 minutes. Both are fine.

If formula feeding: You can give baby a bottle during the first hour or wait until baby shows hunger cues (rooting, sucking on hands, fussiness). Either approach works.

Colostrum: If you're chest-feeding or breastfeeding, your body produces colostrum (thick, yellowish early milk) in small amounts during the first days. This is perfect for newborns—their stomachs are tiny (about the size of a marble), and colostrum provides concentrated nutrients and immune protection.

For non-gestational parents: If you're planning to induce lactation (covered in Chapter 23.0), you can attempt to latch baby even in the first hours. If you're bottle-feeding, you should give some of the first bottles so baby bonds with both parents through feeding from the start.

21.7 Rooming In Versus Nursery

Many hospitals offer rooming-in (baby stays in your room 24/7) or nursery care (baby goes to nursery between feedings). Both options have benefits.

Rooming-in benefits:

- Facilitates bonding

- Allows responsive feeding (feeding on demand rather than schedule)
- Promotes breastfeeding success
- Helps you learn baby's cues
- Keeps family together

Rooming-in challenges:

- Exhausting for parents who just gave birth
- Less sleep (though many parents sleep poorly anyway worrying about baby in nursery)
- More overwhelming for first-time parents

Nursery care benefits:

- Allows rest and recovery
- Nurses monitor baby and bring them for feedings
- Reduces immediate parenting demands

Nursery care drawbacks:

- Less bonding time
- Less responsive feeding
- Baby might receive formula or pacifier without your consent

Most LGBTQ+ families choose: Rooming-in so both parents can be with baby, practice caregiving, and establish feeding. But if you're completely exhausted or had difficult birth, nursery care for a few hours while you sleep is reasonable.

For transgender men: Rooming-in means more exposure to baby-care tasks that might trigger dysphoria. Consider whether having your partner handle most hands-on care while you recover works better for your mental health.

21.8 Going Home After Birth

Hospital stays after vaginal birth typically last 24-48 hours. After cesarean birth, stays are typically 3-4 days.

Before discharge, providers check:

- Your physical recovery (bleeding, pain, ability to urinate)
- Baby's feeding (ensuring baby is eating and not losing too much weight)
- Baby's jaundice levels if applicable
- Baby's bowel movements and urination
- Your emotional wellbeing
- Understanding of warning signs requiring medical attention

What you need at home:

- Place for baby to sleep (bassinet or crib)
- Diapers, wipes, and diaper cream
- Several changes of baby clothes
- Swaddle blankets
- Feeding supplies (bottles and formula if bottle-feeding, nursing pillow if chest-feeding)
- Car seat (properly installed—can't leave hospital without one)

Discharge instructions: Providers give written instructions about baby care, feeding, when to schedule pediatrician appointments, warning signs requiring immediate attention, and postpartum recovery for birthing person.

For LGBTQ+ families: Ensure discharge paperwork includes both parents' names correctly. Check that baby's birth certificate information is accurate regarding parentage. Some hospitals make mistakes with same-sex parents or transgender parents—catch these before leaving.

21.9 Real First Hours Experience

Consider Priya and Nicole's immediate postpartum (composite): Priya gave birth at 9:30pm. Their daughter was placed immediately on Priya's chest. Nicole cut the cord. They both cried, overwhelmed and euphoric.

After 45 minutes of skin-to-skin, the midwife asked if Nicole wanted to hold the baby. Nicole removed her shirt and did skin-to-skin while Priya got stitches for a second-degree tear. Nicole held their daughter for an hour, talking to her, crying, feeling her breathe against her chest.

The baby latched and fed for the first time at 11pm with Priya, then fell asleep. At 2am, she woke hungry. Nicole gave her the second feeding via bottle (pumped colostrum), ensuring both mothers fed their daughter on her first day of life.

They kept their daughter in the room all night despite exhaustion. By morning, they were overwhelmed but deeply in love. Priya's sister came to visit and asked "So who's the real mom?" Both Priya and Nicole said simultaneously: "We both are." Their daughter had two mothers from minute one.

21.10 Essential First Hours Points

The immediate postpartum hours involve skin-to-skin contact with baby, placenta delivery, potential perineal repair, newborn procedures, partner bonding time, first feeding attempts, and decisions about rooming-in versus nursery care. Skin-to-skin contact provides significant benefits for temperature regulation, bonding, and feeding initiation.

For LGBTQ+ families, ensuring both parents get holding and skin-to-skin time establishes equal parenthood from the start. Transgender men and non-binary people can modify skin-to-skin approaches to manage dysphoria while still supporting baby's needs. First feeding attempts happen within the first hour for most babies.

Hospital stays last 24-48 hours after vaginal birth, during which providers monitor recovery and teach basic baby care. Before discharge, ensure birth certificate and hospital paperwork accurately reflect your family structure. The first hours are exhausting, overwhelming, and magical—the beginning of your new life as parents.

Chapter 22.0: The Fourth Trimester

Elena thought she was prepared. She'd read the books, taken the classes, bought all the gear. Then she brought her daughter home and realized nothing prepares you for the reality. The exhaustion was crushing. Her body hurt everywhere. She bled through pads hourly. Her emotions swung wildly—joy, terror, love, resentment, all within minutes. Jasmine kept saying "This is normal, we're doing fine," but Elena felt like she was drowning.

The fourth trimester—the first three months postpartum—is brutally hard. Your body is recovering from birth while you're caring for a completely dependent newborn with no sleep and massive hormonal shifts. This chapter covers physical recovery, hormonal changes, body image and dysphoria, bleeding and healing, when to seek medical attention, postpartum visits, partner experiences, and surviving sleep deprivation.

22.1 Physical Recovery from Birth

Birth is a major physical event requiring significant recovery time, regardless of birth method.

Recovery after vaginal birth:

Perineal healing: If you had tearing or episiotomy, the area will be sore for 1-2 weeks, tender for 2-4 weeks. Ice packs for the first 24-48 hours help. Witch hazel pads, warm sitz baths, and peri bottles (squirt bottles for cleaning after bathroom use) provide relief.

Hemorrhoids: Common after vaginal birth due to pushing. Witch hazel pads, ice packs, and over-the-counter hemorrhoid treatments help. Most resolve within weeks.

Pelvic floor: Muscles are stretched and weakened. Many people experience urinary incontinence (leaking urine when coughing, sneezing, or laughing) for weeks to months postpartum. Pelvic floor physical therapy helps if incontinence persists beyond a few months.

General soreness: Everything hurts—legs, back, arms, abdomen. Rest helps. Gentle movement once you're feeling slightly better also helps.

Recovery after cesarean birth:

Incision care: Keep incision clean and dry. Watch for signs of infection (increased redness, warmth, drainage, fever). Pain at incision site is normal for 1-2 weeks, tenderness for 4-6 weeks.

Abdominal healing: You had major abdominal surgery. Avoid heavy lifting (nothing heavier than baby) for 6 weeks. Don't do abdominal exercises or strenuous activity until cleared by your provider at 6-week checkup.

Getting around: Moving hurts initially. Use pillows to support your incision when standing or moving. Getting in and out of bed is awkward—roll to your side and push up with your arms rather than using abdominal muscles.

Pain management: Take prescribed pain medication as directed. Don't try to tough it out—adequate pain control helps you move more, which speeds recovery.

22.2 Hormonal Changes and Mood

Hormones crash dramatically after birth, causing predictable mood effects.

What happens hormonally: During pregnancy, estrogen and progesterone levels are high. After placenta delivers, these hormones plummet within 24 hours. This sudden drop triggers mood changes in most people.

Baby blues: About 50-80% of people experience "baby blues" in the first two weeks postpartum—tearfulness, mood swings, anxiety, irritability, feeling overwhelmed (American College of Obstetricians and Gynecologists, 2021). This is normal, caused by hormonal shifts, exhaustion, and adjustment. Baby blues typically resolve by two weeks postpartum without treatment.

Postpartum depression: Different from baby blues—more severe, lasts longer, interferes with functioning. We'll cover this fully in Chapter 25.0.

Emotional intensity: Even without baby blues or depression, emotions are intense postpartum. You might cry at commercials, feel sudden rage at small inconveniences, experience overwhelming love, or feel resentment toward your baby or partner within minutes of each other. All normal in the first weeks.

For transgender men: Hormonal shifts might affect you differently since your baseline hormones differ from cisgender women. Stopping testosterone pre-pregnancy already involved hormonal adjustment. Postpartum hormones create another shift. Be especially vigilant about mental health (see Chapter 25.0).

22.3 Body Image and Dysphoria

Postpartum bodies look and feel different than pre-pregnancy bodies. This creates body image challenges for everyone and specific dysphoria for transgender and non-binary people.

Common postpartum body changes:

- Still looking several months pregnant immediately postpartum (uterus takes 6 weeks to shrink back)
- Softer, rounder belly with stretched skin and often stretch marks
- Larger, heavier breasts or chest (especially if chest-feeding)
- Wider hips (pelvis expands during pregnancy)

- Weight retention (most people retain 10-20 pounds for months)
- Loose skin, changed body shape

Body image struggles: Many people struggle with postpartum bodies. Your body did something amazing—grew and birthed a human—but it looks different than before pregnancy, and media tells us bodies should "bounce back" immediately (they don't). Most bodies take 9-12 months to approximate pre-pregnancy shape, and some changes are permanent.

For transgender men and non-binary people: Postpartum dysphoria can be intense. Your body became more feminine-appearing during pregnancy, and some of that persists postpartum. Chest/breast enlargement, wider hips, softer shape—these changes might trigger severe dysphoria.

Managing dysphoria postpartum:

- Plan to resume testosterone as soon as medically appropriate (immediately if not chest-feeding, after weaning if you chest-feed)
- Wear clothes that feel authentic even if they fit differently
- Practice self-compassion—your body did something extraordinary
- Continue therapy for dysphoria management
- Set timeline for body changes you can control (top surgery, resuming testosterone, returning to exercise)
- Remember this is temporary—most changes resolve over months

22.4 Bleeding and Physical Healing

Postpartum bleeding (lochia) is normal and lasts for weeks.

What lochia is: After birth, your uterus sheds the lining that supported pregnancy. This creates bleeding similar to a very heavy period that gradually decreases over 4-6 weeks.

Normal lochia progression:

- First 3-4 days: Heavy red bleeding (soaking through a pad in 2-3 hours is normal)
- Days 4-10: Moderate red to pinkish-brown bleeding
- Days 10-21: Light pink to brown discharge
- Weeks 3-6: Light brownish or yellowish discharge, eventually stopping

Use pads, not tampons: Don't insert anything into your vagina for at least 6 weeks postpartum (risk of infection). Use heavy-duty pads initially, switching to lighter pads as bleeding decreases.

What's concerning:

- Soaking through a pad in one hour
- Passing clots larger than a golf ball
- Foul-smelling discharge (indicates infection)
- Bright red bleeding that returns after turning pink or brown
- Fever with bleeding

Uterine massage: If bleeding is heavy, massaging your uterus (firm rubbing of lower abdomen) helps it contract and reduces bleeding. Nurses teach this in hospital. Chest-feeding or breastfeeding also triggers uterine contractions that reduce bleeding.

22.5 When to Seek Medical Attention

Know warning signs requiring immediate medical attention postpartum.

Emergency warning signs:

- Heavy bleeding (soaking through a pad in one hour or passing large clots)
- Severe abdominal pain (different from normal cramping)
- Fever over 100.4°F
- Severe headache or visual changes

- Chest pain or difficulty breathing
- Severe swelling, redness, or pain in legs (could indicate blood clot)
- Suicidal thoughts or thoughts of harming baby
- Confusion or altered mental state

For cesarean births specifically:

- Increasing incision pain, redness, warmth, or drainage
- Incision opening or separating
- Fever

Don't hesitate: If something feels wrong, call your provider or go to emergency room. Postpartum complications can be serious. Better to get checked and be reassured than to ignore warning signs.

Postpartum preeclampsia: Can develop even after birth, causing high blood pressure, headaches, visual changes, and swelling. This is an emergency requiring immediate treatment (American College of Obstetricians and Gynecologists, 2023).

22.6 Postpartum Visits

Most people have a postpartum checkup at 2 weeks and comprehensive visit at 6 weeks postpartum.

Two-week visit (if offered):

- Brief check of physical recovery
- Assessment of bleeding, pain, healing
- Screening for postpartum depression
- Support for feeding challenges
- Opportunity to ask questions

Six-week visit:

- Physical exam including pelvic exam
- Checking incision healing (if cesarean)

- Blood pressure check
- Depression screening
- Discussion of birth control
- Clearance for exercise and sex
- Addressing any ongoing concerns

What to ask at postpartum visits:

- When can I resume exercise?
- Is my bleeding/pain/healing normal?
- What birth control options work for me?
- How do I manage persistent pain or discomfort?
- I'm struggling emotionally—is this normal or should I be concerned?
- Can I resume testosterone? (for transgender men)

For LGBTQ+ families: Ensure providers recognize your partner's role. If the non-gestational parent has concerns or questions, providers should address them. Don't let providers default to only talking to the birthing person.

22.7 Partner Postpartum Experience

Non-gestational partners also experience postpartum challenges, though different from birthing people's experiences.

Partner exhaustion: You're also sleep-deprived, learning infant care, and adjusting to massive life changes. Non-gestational partners' exhaustion is often dismissed because "you didn't give birth," but caring for a newborn while supporting your partner is genuinely exhausting.

Feeling left out: If your partner is chest-feeding, they spend hours daily feeding the baby while you watch. This can feel isolating. Find other ways to bond—diaper changes, baths, holding and soothing, bottle-feeding if partner pumps.

Relationship strain: Sleep deprivation, stress, and reduced couple time strain relationships. Many couples report relationship satisfaction decreases in the first year postpartum (Doss et al., 2009). This is temporary but real. Maintain communication, express needs directly, and be patient with each other.

Sexual relationship changes: Most providers recommend waiting 6 weeks before resuming sex to allow healing. Many couples wait longer because they're exhausted or the birthing person's body still hurts. This is normal. Don't pressure your partner. Physical intimacy will return.

For non-gestational mothers specifically: Some non-gestational lesbian mothers report feeling like support people rather than co-parents in early weeks, especially if the gestational mother is chest-feeding. Assert your parental status—you're both mothers. Share caregiving equally in domains where you can contribute.

22.8 Sleep Deprivation Survival

Sleep deprivation is one of the hardest parts of early parenthood. Newborns wake every 2-3 hours to eat, giving you at most 90-minute sleep stretches.

How sleep deprivation affects you:

- Cognitive impairment (functioning like you're drunk)
- Emotional dysregulation (crying, irritability, rage)
- Physical exhaustion
- Impaired decision-making
- Increased accident risk

Survival strategies:

Sleep when baby sleeps: Everyone says this. It's actually good advice. Don't use baby's naps to clean or cook—sleep. Dishes can wait.

Take shifts: If two parents are available, take shifts overnight. One person handles 10pm-2am, the other handles 2am-6am. The off-duty parent sleeps in a different room with earplugs. Four-hour sleep blocks feel vastly better than constant interruptions.

Accept help: If people offer help, accept it. Have them hold baby while you nap, bring you food, or do laundry. Don't play martyr.

Lower standards: Your house will be messy. You'll eat takeout. You might not shower daily. All okay. Survival is the goal.

Remember it's temporary: Most babies sleep longer stretches by 8-12 weeks. You won't be this exhausted forever.

For single parents: Sleep deprivation is harder without a partner to share shifts. Can a family member or friend stay with you for the first weeks? Can you hire a postpartum doula for overnight help? Survival requires creative solutions.

22.9 Composite Fourth Trimester

Consider Marcus and Tao's fourth trimester (composite): Marcus gave birth at 39 weeks. For the first two weeks home, he cried daily. His body hurt. He was bleeding heavily. The baby wanted to eat constantly. He felt like he'd never been so tired in his life.

Tao handled most physical baby care initially because Marcus was recovering. But Tao was also exhausted—working from home while caring for baby while supporting Marcus. They snapped at each other over small things. They both cried from exhaustion.

At week three, things got slightly easier. Marcus's bleeding decreased. His incision hurt less. The baby started sleeping in slightly longer chunks. At week six, Marcus resumed testosterone and immediately felt more like himself.

By week eight, they had a rhythm. Still exhausted, still figuring things out, but functional. Marcus's dysphoria decreased as testosterone worked its way back into his system. Their son started smiling, making the exhaustion feel worth it.

By week twelve, the fourth trimester was ending. They felt human again. Their relationship had survived the stress. Their son was thriving. The hardest part was behind them.

22.10 Fourth Trimester Essentials

The fourth trimester involves significant physical recovery from birth, dramatic hormonal shifts causing mood changes, body image challenges and dysphoria for trans/non-binary people, weeks of postpartum bleeding, and crushing sleep deprivation. Recovery after vaginal birth takes 4-6 weeks; after cesarean, 6-8 weeks. Know warning signs requiring immediate medical attention.

Postpartum visits at 2 weeks and 6 weeks monitor recovery and screen for complications. Partners also experience exhaustion, relationship strain, and adjustment challenges. Sleep deprivation affects everyone—take shifts, accept help, and remember it's temporary.

The fourth trimester is the hardest phase of new parenthood. You're healing, hormonally unstable, exhausted, and learning to care for a helpless infant. It gets easier. By 12 weeks, most families have adjusted and feel significantly better. Survive the first months, ask for help, and be gentle with yourself.

Chapter 23.0: Feeding Your Baby

Riley stared at the bottles, the breast pump, the formula cans, the lactation consultant's card, and the Instagram posts about "breast is best." They felt paralyzed. They wanted to chest-feed their baby—it seemed healthiest and most bonding. But chest-feeding triggered severe dysphoria. Formula feeding felt like failure despite knowing rationally it wasn't. Their wife Alex wanted to induce lactation but wasn't sure she could produce enough milk. Three weeks in, they were supplementing with formula, pumping occasionally, attempting to chest-feed sometimes, and feeling like they were failing at everything.

Feeding decisions are loaded with judgment, pressure, and conflicting information. For LGBTQ+ families, feeding involves additional layers: managing dysphoria while chest-feeding, inducing lactation in non-gestational parents, navigating formula feeding without shame, and determining how both parents participate in feeding. This chapter covers all feeding options, combination feeding, pumping, donor milk, partner involvement, and feeding in public as LGBTQ+ families.

23.1 All Feeding Options Are Valid

Let's establish this upfront: however you feed your baby is fine. Chest-feeding, breastfeeding, exclusive pumping, formula feeding, combination feeding—all are valid options that can support healthy babies.

The "breast is best" message: Public health campaigns emphasize breastfeeding benefits—reduced infections, potentially reduced allergy risk, bonding, convenience (no bottles to prepare). These benefits are real but modest. The difference between breastfed and formula-fed babies in developed countries with safe water is small (Grummer-Strawn & Rollins, 2015).

What actually matters: Babies need to be fed, loved, and cared for. The specific method matters far less than adequate nutrition, responsive caregiving, and family wellbeing.

For LGBTQ+ families specifically: Feeding methods that support your mental health, allow both parents to participate, and don't trigger unbearable dysphoria are the right methods. Don't sacrifice your wellbeing for marginal health benefits.

23.2 Chestfeeding for Trans and Non-Binary People

Transgender men and non-binary people can chest-feed if they choose, though this involves complex decisions about dysphoria versus desire to provide milk.

Decision factors:

- How much does chest-feeding trigger dysphoria?
- How important is providing your milk to you?
- Can you manage dysphoria triggers during feeding?
- Do you have support for your decision either way?
- What's your plan for returning to testosterone?

If you choose to chest-feed:

Language: Use terms that feel comfortable—chest-feeding, nursing, feeding, body-feeding. Tell providers and lactation consultants your preferred terms.

Managing dysphoria: Chest-feeding might trigger dysphoria through chest exposure, attention to chest anatomy, and the femininity associated with breastfeeding. Strategies include wearing loose clothing that allows feeding without full exposure, feeding in private rather than in public if that reduces dysphoria, setting time limits on how long you'll chest-feed, and continuing therapy throughout.

Duration decisions: You don't have to chest-feed for a year (the typical recommendation). You can chest-feed for two weeks, six weeks, three months—whatever duration works for you. Stopping when dysphoria becomes unbearable is valid.

Returning to testosterone: You can't chest-feed while on testosterone (it suppresses milk production and passes through milk). If resuming testosterone is important for your mental health, that timeline might determine feeding duration.

If you choose formula:

- Formula feeding is a completely valid choice that doesn't mean you love your baby less
- Your partner can share feeding equally
- You can resume testosterone immediately postpartum
- Your mental health is protected from dysphoria triggers
- Your baby will be healthy and loved

23.3 Induced Lactation

Non-gestational parents can induce lactation to feed their babies, though this requires advance planning and realistic expectations.

How induced lactation works: Milk production is triggered by hormones (estrogen, progesterone, prolactin) and stimulation of breast tissue. Non-pregnant people can mimic these hormonal changes through medications and stimulate milk production through pumping.

The Newman-Goldfarb Protocol: The most established protocol for induced lactation involves birth control pills containing estrogen and progesterone taken continuously for months, plus domperidone (a medication that increases prolactin and milk production—not FDA approved in the U.S. but available in Canada and other countries). Six weeks before baby's arrival, stop birth control and begin regular pumping to stimulate milk production (Goldfarb & Newman, 2019).

Realistic expectations: Most people who induce lactation produce some milk, but many don't produce full supply. You might produce enough for exclusive feeding, or you might produce supplemental amounts requiring formula supplementation. Both outcomes are successful.

Timeline: Starting the protocol 6-12 months before baby's birth gives best results. Shorter timelines are possible but typically produce less milk.

Challenges:

- Time commitment (pumping every 2-3 hours for months)
- Cost of medications and pumping equipment
- Medication side effects
- Uncertainty about how much milk you'll produce
- Emotional investment in something that might not work fully

Benefits:

- Both parents can feed baby breast milk
- Non-gestational parent gets feeding bonding
- Some families find it meaningful for both mothers to provide milk

23.4 Formula Feeding Without Shame

Formula feeding works. Billions of babies have been raised on formula and turned out fine. But formula feeding parents often face judgment and shame.

Formula is safe and nutritious: Modern infant formula is carefully regulated and nutritionally complete. Formula-fed babies grow and develop normally. The health differences between breastfed and formula-fed babies in developed countries are minimal (Grummer-Strawn & Rollins, 2015).

Why formula feeding might be right:

- Chest-feeding triggers severe dysphoria
- Medical conditions preventing chest-feeding
- Medications incompatible with chest-feeding
- Adoption or surrogacy (without induced lactation)
- Personal preference
- Shared feeding between parents
- Previous traumatic experiences with breastfeeding

Handling judgment: People will ask why you're not breastfeeding. Responses: "Formula works great for our family." "We made the choice that's best for us." "That's personal." You don't owe explanations.

Formula feeding logistics:

- Choose a formula (name brands and generic are nutritionally equivalent)
- Prepare bottles according to package directions
- Warm if baby prefers (not required—room temperature is fine)
- Feed responsively (watch baby's cues, not clock)
- Hold baby close during feeding to promote bonding

For LGBTQ+ families: Formula feeding allows both parents equal participation in feeding. Neither parent has biological advantage. This can reduce non-gestational parent feelings of being left out.

23.5 Combination Feeding Strategies

Many families use combination feeding—some breast milk or chest milk, some formula. This allows benefits of each method.

Why combination feeding:

- Chest-feeding parent can't or doesn't want to exclusively chest-feed
- Non-gestational parent wants to participate in feeding
- Return to work makes exclusive chest-feeding difficult
- Inadequate milk supply requiring supplementation
- Managing dysphoria by limiting chest-feeding frequency

How to combination feed:

- Establish chest-feeding or breastfeeding first (2-4 weeks), then introduce bottles
- Feed from chest/breast for some feedings, bottle for others
- Allow non-gestational parent to give bottles
- Use paced bottle feeding (slowing flow to mimic breast)
- Accept that milk supply might decrease with less frequent chest-feeding

Combination feeding and milk supply: Milk production works on supply-and-demand—less feeding means less milk production. If you want to maintain supply while combination feeding, pump when giving bottles instead of nursing.

23.6 Pumping and Bottle Feeding

Exclusively pumping (providing breast milk via bottle rather than direct feeding) works for some families, particularly when chest-feeding triggers dysphoria but parents want baby to receive their milk.

Why exclusive pumping:

- Chest-feeding triggers dysphoria but you want to provide milk
- Baby has difficulty latching
- Need to track exact intake amounts (medical reasons)
- Allows both parents equal feeding participation
- Returning to work

Exclusive pumping logistics:

- Pump every 2-3 hours initially to establish supply (including overnight)
- Pump 15-20 minutes per session
- Store milk in refrigerator (up to 4 days) or freezer (up to 6 months)
- Warm bottles by running under warm water or using bottle warmer
- Both parents can feed from bottles

Challenges:

- Time-consuming (pumping takes as long as feeding)
- Pump maintenance and sterilization
- Harder to maintain supply than direct feeding
- Less convenient when away from home

Benefits:

- Non-gestational parent fully participates in feeding
- Reduced dysphoria compared to chest-feeding
- Tracking exact intake
- Freedom to be away from baby without feeding concerns

23.7 Donor Milk Options

Some families use donor human milk from milk banks or peer-to-peer milk sharing.

Milk banks: Nonprofit milk banks screen donors medically, pasteurize milk, and distribute to babies who need it (primarily premature babies or babies with medical conditions). Banked donor milk is safest donor milk option but expensive and often limited availability (Human Milk Banking Association of North America, 2023).

Peer milk sharing: Some parents share milk informally through online communities (Human Milk 4 Human Babies, Eats on Feets). This is less expensive but carries risks since milk isn't screened or pasteurized. Donors might have infections or take medications passing through milk.

Why donor milk:

- Want baby to receive human milk but can't provide it yourself
- Inadequate supply requiring supplementation
- Adoption or surrogacy

Considerations: Donor milk is generally safe if from screened, healthy donors, but risks exist with informal milk sharing. Weigh benefits against risks and costs.

23.8 Partner Involvement in Feeding

Both parents should participate in feeding regardless of method.

If chest-feeding or breastfeeding:

- Non-feeding parent handles diaper changes, burping, holding after feeds
- Give bottles of pumped milk or formula occasionally so non-feeding parent does full feeding
- Non-feeding parent takes overnight shifts when possible (bring baby to feeding parent for feeding, then handle everything else)
- Split other caregiving tasks equally to balance feeding parent's time investment

If formula feeding or exclusively pumping:

- Take turns with feedings—alternate who feeds for each feeding or split day into shifts

- One parent handles night feedings one night, other parent handles next night
- Both parents do equal diaper changes, soothing, and other care

Importance of equal involvement: Non-gestational parents who actively participate in feeding and caregiving bond more securely with babies and report better co-parenting relationships (Fillo et al., 2015).

23.9 Feeding in Public

Feeding babies in public spaces sometimes creates discomfort, especially for LGBTQ+ families.

Legal protections: In the U.S., breastfeeding is legally protected in all 50 states—you can breastfeed or chest-feed anywhere you're legally allowed to be. But legal protection doesn't prevent stares or comments.

For transgender men chest-feeding in public: You might be read as male, making public chest-feeding even more gender-transgressive. This can attract stares, comments, or harassment. Strategies include feeding in private spaces (car, nursing rooms, bathroom stalls), using nursing covers if that helps, choosing LGBTQ+-friendly locations when possible, or having your partner present as buffer against harassment.

For lesbian couples: Public feeding rarely causes issues beyond standard breastfeeding reactions. But if one mother is feeding the baby and the other is obviously her partner, you might get questions or stares about your family structure.

For all LGBTQ+ families with formula: Formula feeding in public generally attracts less attention than breastfeeding, though some people might ask invasive questions about why you're not breastfeeding. Responses: "Formula works for us." You don't owe explanations.

23.10 Your Feeding Decision

Consider this decision framework for your family:

Questions to ask:

- What matters most to us—providing our milk, equal parent participation, protecting mental health, convenience?
- Can the gestational parent chest-feed without severe dysphoria? For how long?
- Does the non-gestational parent want to induce lactation?
- What feeding method allows both parents meaningful involvement?
- What's sustainable long-term given work, mental health, and family needs?

Make decisions that work for your specific family. Revisit decisions as circumstances change—you can start with one method and switch if it's not working.

23.11 Core Feeding Principles

All feeding methods—chest-feeding, breastfeeding, induced lactation, formula feeding, combination feeding, exclusive pumping—support healthy babies. For transgender and non-binary people, feeding decisions involve balancing desire to provide milk against dysphoria triggers. Non-gestational parents can induce lactation with realistic expectations about milk production.

Formula feeding is safe, nutritious, and valid—don't let shame influence your decision. Combination feeding allows benefits of multiple methods. Exclusive pumping provides breast milk via bottle, reducing dysphoria while maintaining milk supply. Both parents should actively participate in feeding regardless of method.

The right feeding method is the one that supports your baby's nutrition, your mental health, both parents' involvement, and your family's wellbeing. There's no single right answer—just the answer that works for your specific situation.

Chapter 24.0: Chestfeeding and Lactation

Maria latched her daughter for the first time and felt... nothing like she expected. The baby's mouth felt weird on her nipple. It didn't hurt exactly, but it was uncomfortable and strange. Everyone talked about bonding and oxytocin and this magical connection, but mostly Maria felt awkward and wondered if she was doing it wrong. By day three, her nipples were cracked and bleeding. By week two, she'd figured out positioning and the pain had resolved. By week six, feeding felt natural and even enjoyable. But those first weeks were hard in ways nobody had warned her about.

Chestfeeding and breastfeeding aren't instinctive or automatic for most people. They're learned skills requiring practice, problem-solving, and often support. This chapter covers how lactation works, initiating milk production, positioning and latch, common challenges and solutions, chestfeeding after top surgery, medications and safety, managing dysphoria, and weaning. If you're planning to chest-feed or breastfeed, this is your detailed guide.

24.1 How Lactation Works

Understanding the biology of milk production helps you troubleshoot problems and maintain supply.

Hormonal control: During pregnancy, estrogen and progesterone are high, preparing breast/chest tissue for lactation but preventing actual milk production. After placenta delivery, these hormones drop dramatically, triggering milk production through the hormone prolactin.

Colostrum: For the first 2-4 days postpartum, you produce colostrum—thick, yellowish early milk in small amounts (typically

2-20 ml per feeding). This is exactly right for newborns whose stomachs are tiny. Colostrum is concentrated with nutrients, antibodies, and immune factors.

Milk "coming in": Around days 3-5 postpartum, your mature milk production increases dramatically. Your breasts or chest become engorged (full, hard, sometimes painful). This is when milk volume increases from milliliters to ounces per feeding.

Supply and demand: Milk production is driven by how much milk is removed. More frequent feeding or pumping signals your body to produce more milk. Less frequent removal decreases supply. This means supply adjusts to baby's needs over time.

Let-down reflex: When baby latches or you pump, oxytocin causes milk to "let down"—flow from the milk-producing glands. You might feel tingling, warmth, or sudden fullness when this happens. Multiple let-downs can occur during one feeding.

For transgender men and non-binary people: Your chest tissue functions the same way as cisgender women's breast tissue for lactation purposes if you haven't had top surgery. Testosterone doesn't prevent lactation—stopping testosterone allows lactation to occur normally in most cases.

24.2 Initiating Milk Production

The first days of feeding establish your milk supply and help baby learn to feed effectively.

Skin-to-skin and early feeding: Immediate skin-to-skin contact after birth and early feeding attempts (within the first hour) support successful feeding initiation. Even if baby doesn't latch immediately, the skin-to-skin contact and practice attempts help (Moore et al., 2016).

Frequent feeding: Newborns typically feed 8-12 times per 24 hours (every 2-3 hours). This frequent feeding stimulates milk production and prevents engorgement. Don't try to space out feedings or implement schedules in early weeks—feed on demand.

Both breasts or one? Some babies feed from both breasts each feeding, others from one breast per feeding. Either pattern works. Follow baby's cues—when they release one side and seem content, offer the other side. If they refuse, that's fine.

Night feeding: Night feedings are essential for maintaining supply and for baby's nutrition. Prolactin levels are higher at night, making night feedings especially important for milk production. Don't skip them.

Watch baby, not the clock: Feed when baby shows hunger cues (rooting, sucking on hands, fussiness)—don't wait for crying (late hunger cue). Feed until baby releases the breast/chest and seems satisfied, not for a predetermined number of minutes.

Engorgement management: When milk comes in, your breasts or chest might become painfully engorged. Feed frequently, use cold compresses between feedings, take ibuprofen for pain, and hand-express a small amount before feeding if engorgement makes it hard for baby to latch.

24.3 Positioning and Latch

Proper positioning and latch are crucial for comfortable, effective feeding and preventing nipple damage.

Good latch characteristics:

- Baby's mouth opens wide before latching
- Baby takes in significant breast/chest tissue (not just nipple)
- Baby's lips flange outward
- You see more areola visible above baby's top lip than below bottom lip
- Baby's cheeks remain rounded (not sucked in) during feeding

- You hear swallowing but minimal clicking or smacking sounds

Common positions:

Cradle hold: Baby lies across your front, tummy to tummy with you, head in the crook of your arm. Classic position but can be hard for newborns who need more head support.

Cross-cradle hold: Similar to cradle but you hold baby's head with the hand opposite the breast/chest they're feeding from. Gives more control for positioning newborns.

Football hold: Baby lies along your side, feet toward your back, head cradled in your hand. Good for cesarean recovery (keeps baby off incision) and for people with large breasts/chest.

Side-lying: You and baby lie on your sides facing each other. Good for night feedings and cesarean recovery. Requires practice to position safely.

Laid-back or biological nurturing: You recline back at angle, baby lies on your front and self-attaches to breast/chest. Can feel very natural and comfortable.

Achieving good latch: Position baby at breast/chest level (use pillows if needed), wait for baby's mouth to open wide, bring baby to you quickly when mouth opens (don't lean yourself toward baby), ensure baby takes in significant tissue. If it hurts beyond the first few seconds, unlatch (insert finger to break suction) and try again.

24.4 Common Challenges and Solutions

Most people encounter challenges with chestfeeding or breastfeeding. Solutions exist for nearly all of them.

Sore nipples: Some initial tenderness is normal in first week. But cracked, bleeding, or severely painful nipples indicate latch problems. Solutions: improve latch (watch videos or work with lactation consultant), use nipple cream (purified lanolin or coconut oil), let nipples air dry after feeding, change breast pads frequently.

Low supply concerns: Many people worry about low supply when supply is actually adequate. Baby's output is the best indicator—6+ wet diapers and 3+ poopy diapers daily by day 5 indicates adequate intake. If supply is genuinely low: feed more frequently, ensure good latch, pump after feedings, increase fluid intake, consider galactagogues (substances that increase milk production—oatmeal, fenugreek, blessed thistle, prescription domperidone where available).

Oversupply: Some people produce too much milk, causing baby to choke, gag, or spit up excessively. Solutions: feed from only one breast per feeding, recline during feeding (gravity slows flow), hand-express small amount before latching to reduce initial fast flow.

Engorgement: Extremely full, hard breasts/chest in first weeks. Solutions: feed frequently, use cold compresses between feedings, hand-express just enough to soften before feeding, take ibuprofen for pain.

Plugged ducts: Localized hard, tender lump in breast/chest from milk backing up in a duct. Solutions: feed frequently, massage affected area toward nipple while feeding, apply warm compresses before feeding, ensure bra isn't too tight.

Mastitis: Infection in breast/chest tissue causing flu-like symptoms (fever, body aches, chills) plus red, hot, painful area. Requires antibiotics. Continue feeding or pumping to clear infection—stopping makes it worse. Contact provider if you suspect mastitis.

Tongue-tie or lip-tie: Restricted frenulum (tissue under tongue or lip) can prevent good latch. If suspected, consult pediatric dentist or ENT for evaluation. Some ties require surgical release for effective feeding.

Working with lactation consultants: International Board Certified Lactation Consultants (IBCLCs) specialize in solving feeding problems. Seek help early if struggling—don't wait until problems are severe. Many insurances cover lactation consultation.

24.5 Chestfeeding After Top Surgery

Transgender men and non-binary people who've had top surgery before pregnancy cannot chestfeed (mammary tissue is removed during surgery). But if pregnancy occurs before top surgery, chestfeeding is possible.

Post-surgery considerations: Different top surgery techniques affect future lactation capacity differently:

Double incision mastectomy: Removes most mammary tissue and repositions nipples. This usually eliminates or severely reduces lactation capacity. Some tissue might remain that could produce small amounts of milk, but exclusive chestfeeding is unlikely.

Peri-areolar or keyhole techniques: Remove less tissue and maintain nipple attachment. These preserve more lactation capacity, though milk production might still be reduced compared to no surgery.

Planning considerations: If you know you want biological children eventually and might want to chestfeed, discuss timing of top surgery with your surgeon. Some transgender men choose to delay top surgery until after they've completed family building. Others prioritize top surgery for mental health and accept that chestfeeding won't be possible. Both decisions are valid.

Alternatives after top surgery: If you've had top surgery and want baby to receive your milk, pumping from remaining tissue might produce small amounts that can be supplemented with formula. Or you can exclusively formula-feed, which works perfectly well.

24.6 Medications and Safety

Many medications are compatible with chestfeeding or breastfeeding, but some aren't.

Generally safe medications:

- Most antibiotics
- Acetaminophen (Tylenol) and ibuprofen (Advil, Motrin)
- Most antidepressants (SSRIs like sertraline and fluoxetine)
- Birth control pills containing only progestin (estrogen can reduce supply)
- Most common prescription medications

Medications requiring caution or avoidance:

- Some antidepressants and anti-anxiety medications (discuss with provider)
- Stimulant medications for ADHD (might reduce supply or pass to baby)
- Some pain medications (opioids pass through milk—use as prescribed for short-term only)
- Testosterone (incompatible with lactation—suppresses milk production and passes through milk)

Checking medication safety: LactMed (database from National Library of Medicine) and Infant Risk Center hotline (806-352-2519) provide evidence-based information about medication safety during lactation.

For transgender men: If you're taking testosterone, you cannot chestfeed. Testosterone suppresses milk production and passes through milk to baby. If you want to chestfeed, you must remain off testosterone throughout the feeding period. This creates difficult timing decisions—how long can you tolerate being off testosterone for dysphoria management?

When to resume testosterone: Once you're finished chestfeeding and have fully weaned, you can resume testosterone immediately. There's no waiting period beyond complete weaning.

24.7 Dysphoria and Body Boundaries

For transgender men and non-binary people, chestfeeding often triggers dysphoria despite choosing to do it.

Common dysphoria triggers during chestfeeding:

- Physical sensation of feeding (mouth on chest)
- Watching baby feed from your chest
- Chest enlargement from milk production
- Leaking milk between feedings
- Gendered language around feeding ("breastfeeding," "nursing mother")
- Public perception when chestfeeding

Managing dysphoria while chestfeeding:

Use preferred language: Call it chestfeeding, body-feeding, nursing, or feeding—whatever feels least gendered to you. Correct people who use "breastfeeding" if that language bothers you.

Set boundaries: You don't have to chestfeed for any predetermined duration. If dysphoria becomes unbearable, wean. Your mental health matters more than marginal health benefits of extended chestfeeding.

Feed privately: If public chestfeeding triggers dysphoria due to visibility, feed at home or in private spaces. Don't force yourself to feed publicly if it's overwhelming.

Time limits: Decide you'll chestfeed for six weeks, three months, whatever duration feels manageable, then wean and resume testosterone. Having an endpoint helps.

Partner support: Your partner can handle other baby care tasks while you handle feeding, balancing the emotional labor. They can also advocate against gendered language that misgenders you.

Therapy: Continue therapy throughout chestfeeding to process dysphoria, celebrate your strength in doing this difficult thing, and prepare for weaning and testosterone resumption.

Permission to stop: You can stop chestfeeding at any time for any reason. Unbearable dysphoria is a valid reason. Your baby will be fine on formula. Protect your mental health.

24.8 Weaning Considerations

Weaning—gradually decreasing and eventually stopping chestfeeding or breastfeeding—can be baby-led, parent-led, or collaborative.

Baby-led weaning: Baby naturally reduces feeding frequency as solid foods are introduced (around 6 months) and eventually self-weans, typically between 1-4 years. This works well if you're comfortable continuing until baby decides to stop.

Parent-led weaning: You decide when to wean based on return to work, resuming medications, personal preferences, or (for transgender men) need to resume testosterone. This involves gradually reducing feeding sessions over weeks to allow supply to decrease without causing engorgement or plugged ducts.

Gradual weaning process:

1. Drop one feeding every 3-5 days
2. Replace dropped feeding with bottle (formula or pumped milk) or solid foods (if baby is old enough)
3. Start with feedings baby seems least interested in
4. Continue until only morning and night feedings remain
5. Finally eliminate those feedings

Abrupt weaning: Sometimes necessary due to medical reasons or urgent need to resume medications. Risks include engorgement, plugged ducts, and mastitis. If you must wean abruptly, pump just enough to relieve pressure (not empty completely), use cold compresses, wear supportive bra, and take ibuprofen for pain.

Emotional aspects: Weaning can trigger unexpected emotions—relief, guilt, sadness, freedom. These coexist. For transgender men, weaning often brings immense relief as it allows testosterone resumption. For others, weaning might bring sadness about ending that phase. Both reactions are normal.

Resuming testosterone after weaning: Wait until weaning is complete and milk production has fully stopped before resuming testosterone. This ensures any remaining milk doesn't stay trapped in chest tissue causing problems.

24.9 Real Chestfeeding Experience

Consider Kai's chestfeeding journey (composite): Kai, a transgender man, chose to chestfeed despite knowing it would trigger dysphoria. He wanted to give his son the immune benefits of his milk, and he felt it was something his male body could do that others couldn't.

The first two weeks were physically painful—cracked nipples, engorgement, difficulty getting his son to latch. By week three, the physical pain resolved and feeding became comfortable. But the dysphoria increased. Watching his son feed from his chest triggered feelings of being female that he hadn't felt in years.

Kai used exclusively masculine language—chestfeeding, nursing, feeding his son—and corrected anyone who said "breastfeeding." He fed only at home, refusing to feed in public because he couldn't bear the thought of being perceived as a woman nursing a baby.

He set a goal: six weeks of exclusive chestfeeding, then gradual weaning. At week six, he introduced bottles of formula. By week ten, he was down to morning and bedtime feeds. At week twelve, he fully weaned. Within three days, milk production stopped. He resumed testosterone immediately.

Looking back, Kai felt proud that he'd chestfed for three months despite the dysphoria, but also relieved when it was over. His son had received his milk, and he could return to testosterone and feel like himself again. The decision to chestfeed was right for him, but so was the decision to wean when he did.

24.10 Essential Lactation Knowledge

Lactation works through supply-and-demand—frequent milk removal stimulates production. Colostrum in the first days transitions to mature milk around days 3-5. Proper positioning and deep latch are crucial for comfortable, effective feeding. Common challenges like sore nipples, supply concerns, and engorgement have solutions.

Transgender men who've had top surgery cannot chestfeed due to removed mammary tissue. Timing of top surgery relative to family building involves weighing mental health benefits against potential desire to chestfeed. Most medications are compatible with lactation, but testosterone is not—chestfeeding requires staying off testosterone throughout.

Chestfeeding as a transgender man involves managing significant dysphoria. Setting boundaries, using preferred language, feeding privately, and establishing endpoint timelines help. Permission to stop when dysphoria becomes unbearable is valid. Weaning can be gradual or abrupt depending on circumstances, allowing testosterone resumption once complete.

Chapter 25.0: Postpartum Mental Health

Riley couldn't stop checking if the baby was breathing. Every ten minutes, they'd wake from whatever half-sleep they'd managed and lean over the bassinet to watch their daughter's chest rise and fall. If they couldn't see movement immediately, panic flooded their body—heart racing, sweating, convinced their daughter had stopped breathing. This happened 30, 40 times a night. Their wife Alex begged them to sleep, but Riley couldn't. The anxiety was consuming them.

Postpartum mental health problems affect up to 20% of new parents—depression, anxiety, obsessive-compulsive symptoms, and rarely psychosis. For LGBTQ+ people, rates might be higher due to additional stressors including dysphoria, discrimination, and lack of support. This chapter covers baby blues versus postpartum depression, postpartum anxiety and OCD, postpartum psychosis, birth trauma and PTSD, non-gestational partner mental health, dysphoria intensification, when to seek help, and medication safety.

25.1 Baby Blues Versus Depression

Understanding the difference between temporary baby blues and clinical postpartum depression is crucial.

Baby blues:

- Affects 50-80% of postpartum people
- Begins within first few days postpartum
- Symptoms include tearfulness, mood swings, irritability, anxiety, feeling overwhelmed
- Peaks around day 5, resolves by two weeks postpartum
- Caused by hormonal shifts, exhaustion, adjustment

- Doesn't require treatment—resolves on its own with support and rest

Postpartum depression (PPD):

- Affects 10-15% of postpartum people (Dennis et al., 2017)
- Can begin any time in first year postpartum (often weeks 2-12)
- Symptoms include persistent sadness, hopelessness, loss of interest in activities, difficulty bonding with baby, intrusive thoughts, changes in sleep or appetite, difficulty concentrating, thoughts of death or suicide
- Doesn't resolve on its own—requires treatment
- Not caused by anything you did wrong—results from hormonal changes, genetic vulnerability, stress, and other factors

Key differences: Baby blues resolve within two weeks. Postpartum depression persists, worsens, or begins after the two-week mark. Baby blues involve mood swings and crying. PPD involves persistent low mood, hopelessness, and impaired functioning.

Screening: Providers should screen for PPD at postpartum visits using validated tools like the Edinburgh Postnatal Depression Scale. If you score high or have concerning symptoms, your provider should refer you for mental health treatment.

25.2 Postpartum Anxiety and OCD

Anxiety disorders are actually more common than depression in the postpartum period but receive less attention.

Postpartum anxiety: Characterized by excessive worry, racing thoughts, physical symptoms (heart racing, difficulty breathing, nausea), difficulty sleeping even when baby sleeps, sense of dread, feeling like something bad will happen. Anxiety often focuses on baby's health and safety—obsessive checking, inability to let others care for baby, catastrophic thinking about potential harm.

Postpartum OCD: Involves intrusive thoughts (unwanted, disturbing thoughts that pop into your head) often about harming the baby, plus compulsive behaviors to reduce anxiety from those thoughts. The thoughts are ego-dystonic (distressing to you—you don't want them and wouldn't act on them) but feel uncontrollable (Fairbrother et al., 2016).

Common intrusive thoughts: Thoughts of dropping baby, baby suffocating, accidentally hurting baby, intentionally harming baby. These thoughts are common (up to 90% of new parents have occasional intrusive thoughts), but in postpartum OCD they're frequent, distressing, and lead to compulsive checking or avoidance behaviors.

Distinguishing OCD from psychosis: In postpartum OCD, you recognize the thoughts as wrong and distressing—you don't want to harm your baby and won't. In postpartum psychosis (very rare), you might believe the thoughts are commands or not recognize them as problematic. OCD is much more common than psychosis.

Treatment: Therapy (particularly exposure and response prevention, a type of CBT) and medications (SSRIs) both effectively treat postpartum anxiety and OCD.

25.3 Postpartum Psychosis Warning Signs

Postpartum psychosis is rare (1-2 per 1,000 births) but a psychiatric emergency requiring immediate treatment (VanderKruik et al., 2017).

Symptoms:

- Confusion or disorientation
- Hallucinations (seeing or hearing things that aren't there)
- Delusions (fixed false beliefs)
- Severe mood swings (extreme highs and lows)
- Paranoia
- Disorganized thinking or behavior

- Thoughts of harming yourself or baby

Risk factors: Previous psychosis, bipolar disorder, previous postpartum psychosis, family history of bipolar disorder or psychosis.

Onset: Usually begins within first two weeks postpartum, often within first 48-72 hours.

Treatment: Postpartum psychosis requires immediate psychiatric hospitalization. It's treated with antipsychotic medications, mood stabilizers, and close monitoring. With proper treatment, most people recover fully.

If you or your partner show signs: Go to emergency room immediately or call 911. Postpartum psychosis is dangerous without treatment but responds well to appropriate care.

25.4 PTSD from Birth Trauma

Some people develop post-traumatic stress disorder following traumatic birth experiences.

What constitutes birth trauma: Trauma is subjective—what feels traumatic to one person might not to another. Potentially traumatic birth experiences include emergency cesarean, severe pain, feeling loss of control, feeling disrespected or violated by providers, complications threatening your or baby's life, extensive medical interventions, or NICU admission (Ayers et al., 2016).

PTSD symptoms postpartum:

- Intrusive memories or flashbacks of birth
- Nightmares about birth
- Avoiding thinking or talking about birth
- Hypervigilance and startle responses
- Difficulty bonding with baby (baby triggers memories of trauma)

- Emotional numbness
- Anger or irritability

For transgender men: Birth might be inherently traumatic due to dysphoria, exposure, misgendering during labor, or the trauma of giving birth while male. Even "uncomplicated" births can be traumatic when they involved discrimination or intense dysphoria.

Treatment: Trauma-focused therapy (EMDR or trauma-focused CBT) effectively treats birth-related PTSD. Processing the trauma with a trained therapist helps reduce symptoms and improve bonding with baby.

25.5 Non-Gestational Partner Mental Health

Non-gestational partners also experience postpartum mental health problems, though these are under-recognized.

Postpartum depression in non-gestational partners: About 10% of non-gestational partners experience PPD (Paulson & Bazemore, 2010). Symptoms are similar to gestational parent PPD—persistent sadness, loss of interest, difficulty bonding with baby, feeling inadequate as a parent, hopelessness.

Risk factors for partner PPD: Partner's depression (it's often contagious within couples), sleep deprivation, relationship strain, feeling left out of parent-baby bond, lack of social support, financial stress.

Postpartum anxiety in partners: Non-gestational partners often experience severe anxiety about baby's wellbeing, financial security, their ability to parent, or their relationship surviving the transition.

Why partner mental health matters: Partner mental health affects family functioning, co-parenting quality, and baby's development. Untreated partner depression predicts relationship problems and parenting difficulties. Partners need and deserve mental health support.

Barriers to getting help: Non-gestational partners often don't recognize their symptoms as postpartum mental health problems (they think these only affect birthing people). They might not have access to screening at medical appointments. They might feel they don't deserve help since they "didn't give birth."

What partners need: Screening for depression and anxiety, access to mental health care, recognition that their struggles are real and treatable, partner support from their co-parent.

25.6 Dysphoria Intensification Postpartum

For transgender men and non-binary people, dysphoria often intensifies in the postpartum period beyond pregnancy levels.

Why dysphoria worsens postpartum:

- Body still looks pregnant for weeks postpartum
- If chestfeeding, chest is larger and more feminine-appearing
- Still off testosterone if chestfeeding
- Postpartum bleeding feels like menstruation
- Postpartum hormones are intensely feminizing
- Exhaustion reduces capacity to cope with dysphoria
- Constant misgendering in medical settings and public spaces

Dysphoria versus depression: Dysphoria and depression can coexist and can look similar (both involve distress, mood changes, difficulty functioning). But dysphoria is distress specifically about gender and body, while depression is more generalized mood disturbance. Treatment differs—dysphoria responds to gender-affirming interventions (resuming testosterone, binding, preferred language), while depression requires therapy and possibly medication.

Managing postpartum dysphoria:

- Resume testosterone as soon as medically appropriate (immediately if not chestfeeding, after weaning if chestfeeding)
- Return to binding as soon as medically safe (after cesarean healing or once chestfeeding ends)
- Use masculine clothing even if nothing fits perfectly
- Insist on correct pronouns with all providers
- Continue therapy focused on dysphoria management
- Connect with other trans men who've been through postpartum

When dysphoria triggers depression: Severe, unmanaged dysphoria can trigger depression. If you're experiencing both, treat both—gender-affirming care plus mental health treatment.

25.7 When and How to Seek Help

Knowing when to seek professional mental health support and how to access it is crucial.

When to seek help:

- Symptoms persist beyond two weeks postpartum
- Symptoms interfere with functioning (can't care for baby, can't complete basic tasks)
- Thoughts of harming yourself or baby
- Severe anxiety preventing sleep even when baby sleeps
- Intrusive thoughts that won't stop
- Feeling detached from baby or lacking affection for baby
- Feeling hopeless or like your family would be better off without you
- Substance use to cope

Who to contact:

- Your prenatal care provider (midwife or OB) at postpartum visits
- Your primary care physician

- Therapist specializing in perinatal mental health
- Psychiatrist for medication evaluation
- Postpartum Support International warmline: 1-800-944-4773
- Crisis lines if you're in immediate danger

Types of treatment:

Therapy: Individual therapy (CBT, IPT, psychodynamic therapy) addresses thoughts, behaviors, and coping. Group therapy provides peer support. Both effectively treat postpartum mental health conditions (Sockol, 2015).

Medication: Many psychiatric medications are safe during lactation. SSRIs (sertraline, fluoxetine) are first-line for postpartum depression and anxiety. Medications begin working in 2-4 weeks.

Intensive programs: Some areas offer intensive outpatient programs for perinatal mental health, allowing treatment while staying home with baby. A few programs offer residential treatment for severe postpartum mental health crises.

Don't wait: Early treatment prevents worsening. If you're struggling, seek help now—don't wait to see if it resolves on its own.

25.8 Medications Compatible with Feeding

Many psychiatric medications are compatible with chestfeeding or breastfeeding, allowing treatment without requiring weaning.

Generally compatible medications:

- Sertraline (Zoloft)—first-choice SSRI for lactation
- Fluoxetine (Prozac)
- Paroxetine (Paxil)
- Nortriptyline (tricyclic antidepressant)
- Many anti-anxiety medications

Medications requiring more caution: Some medications pass through milk in higher amounts or affect babies more. Discuss risks and benefits with providers. Often benefits of treating your mental health outweigh small risks of medication exposure through milk.

If you're not feeding: All psychiatric medications are options. You can choose based on effectiveness without lactation concerns.

Decision-making: Work with a provider knowledgeable about psychiatric medications and lactation. Resources like LactMed and Infant Risk Center provide evidence-based guidance. Don't suffer unnecessarily—many treatment options exist.

25.9 Composite Mental Health Journey

Consider Elena and Jasmine's experience (composite): Elena gave birth at 38 weeks. The first week felt overwhelming but manageable. By week three, Elena couldn't stop crying. She felt detached from her daughter. She had intrusive thoughts about something terrible happening to the baby. She couldn't sleep even when the baby slept.

Jasmine recognized Elena was struggling beyond normal adjustment. At the four-week pediatrician appointment, Jasmine privately told the pediatrician "I think my wife has postpartum depression." The pediatrician had Elena complete depression screening, which scored high for PPD.

Elena started therapy immediately with a perinatal mental health specialist and began sertraline (safe while breastfeeding). Within two weeks, Elena felt slightly better. By six weeks, she felt significantly better—more connected to her daughter, less anxious, sleeping better, crying less.

Jasmine also struggled with anxiety and feeling inadequate as a parent, but didn't recognize it as PPD initially. At three months postpartum, Elena encouraged Jasmine to see a therapist. Jasmine started therapy and learned coping strategies for her anxiety.

By six months postpartum, both mothers felt significantly better. They'd survived the hardest part with professional help, medication, therapy, and mutual support. Their mental health struggles were real, but they were also treatable. Getting help early made all the difference.

25.10 Core Mental Health Principles

Postpartum mental health problems are common, affecting 15-20% of birthing people and 10% of non-gestational partners. Baby blues resolve within two weeks; postpartum depression persists and requires treatment. Postpartum anxiety and OCD involve excessive worry and intrusive thoughts. Postpartum psychosis is rare but a psychiatric emergency.

Birth trauma can cause PTSD requiring specialized trauma treatment. Non-gestational partners also experience depression and anxiety deserving recognition and treatment. For transgender men, dysphoria often intensifies postpartum, potentially triggering or worsening depression.

Seek help when symptoms persist beyond two weeks, interfere with functioning, or involve thoughts of self-harm. Treatment includes therapy, medication (many compatible with feeding), and intensive programs. Early intervention prevents worsening and supports family wellbeing. Your mental health matters as much as your baby's wellbeing.

Chapter 26.0: Navigating Newborn Care

Priya and Nicole brought their daughter home from the hospital and realized they had no idea what they were doing. They'd taken infant care classes, but a plastic doll is very different from a screaming, squirming, real baby. The pediatrician asked at the two-day appointment "So how are mothers doing?" and both Priya and Nicole simultaneously said "We're both mothers." The pediatrician apologized and corrected. By the two-week appointment, the entire staff knew their family structure and treated both mothers equally.

Newborn care as LGBTQ+ parents involves the same practical tasks as any parents—feeding, diapering, soothing—plus navigating medical systems that often don't recognize your family structure, making legal parentage decisions, explaining your family to providers, and dividing labor equitably. This chapter covers pediatrician selection, birth certificates and legal parentage, explaining your family, newborn care basics, partner equity, managing visitors, and building your support village.

26.1 Pediatrician Selection and Advocacy

Choosing a pediatrician who respects your family matters enormously for your experience over the next 18 years.

Finding LGBTQ+ affirming pediatricians: Look for pediatricians who advertise LGBTQ+ family competency on their website, ask for recommendations from other LGBTQ+ parents, check reviews specifically mentioning same-sex or transgender parents, and interview potential pediatricians before birth or during first weeks postpartum.

Questions to ask potential pediatricians:

- How many LGBTQ+ families do you serve?
- How do you document multiple mothers, two fathers, or transgender parents in your system?
- How do you ensure all parents receive medical information and participate in decisions?
- What's your experience with non-biological parents' rights?
- How do you handle pronoun use for transgender parents?
- What do your intake forms look like? (Ask to see one)

Red flags:

- Visible discomfort or surprise at your family structure
- Asking invasive questions about conception ("So who's the biological mother?")
- Defaulting to only talking to the gestational parent
- Forms that only have space for "mother" and "father"
- Staff repeatedly misgendering you despite corrections

What affirming care looks like: Forms with "Parent 1" and "Parent 2" rather than "Mother" and "Father," staff using both parents' names naturally, directing information to both parents equally, respecting pronouns without surprise or difficulty, matter-of-fact treatment of your family as normal.

Switching pediatricians: If your pediatrician isn't affirming, switch. You'll be seeing pediatricians frequently for years—don't stay with someone who makes you uncomfortable or fails to recognize your family.

26.2 Birth Certificates and Legal Parentage

Establishing legal parentage for both parents is crucial and varies by location.

Birth certificates: In most states, the birthing person is automatically listed as parent on the birth certificate. The second parent's status varies:

For married same-sex couples: Many states now allow both mothers' or both fathers' names on birth certificates if married. But some states still resist this. Check your state's requirements.

For unmarried same-sex couples: Second-parent adoption is typically required to establish legal parentage.

For transgender men: Some states list you as "mother" despite being male, requiring court action to change to "father." Others allow "father" designation if you request it. Know your state's policies.

Correcting birth certificates: If your birth certificate is issued incorrectly (wrong parent names, wrong gender designations, etc.), you can file corrections. This might require working with hospital vital records office and state vital statistics office. Don't accept incorrect birth certificates—fix them immediately.

Second-parent adoption: Most states require the non-biological parent in same-sex couples to complete second-parent adoption to establish legal parentage, even if you're married. This typically involves:

- Filing petition with court
- Home study (sometimes required, sometimes waived)
- Final court hearing establishing legal parentage
- Updated birth certificate listing both parents

Start this process early postpartum. Consult with LGBTQ+ family law attorneys to understand your state's specific requirements.

Why legal parentage matters: Without legal parentage, the non-biological parent has no legal rights to make medical decisions, no automatic custody if relationship ends, no rights if biological parent dies, and might face challenges with school enrollment or travel. Legal parentage protects your family.

26.3 Explaining Your Family

You'll explain your family structure repeatedly—to pediatricians, other parents, strangers who comment on your baby, family members, eventually your child.

Scripts for explaining:

For lesbian couples: "We're both her mothers." "She has two moms." "We used a donor." Keep it simple unless people need more information.

For gay couples using surrogacy: "We used a surrogate." "A woman carried our baby for us." "We're both his fathers."

For transgender men: "Yes, I'm the father. Yes, I gave birth. Transgender men can become pregnant."

For non-binary parents: "I'm their parent." Use whatever parental terms feel right—parent, ren, dad, something else. Explain if people seem confused, but don't over-explain.

For polyamorous or co-parenting families: "She has three parents." "We're co-parenting our child together." You don't owe details about your romantic or sexual relationships.

Handling invasive questions: People will ask nosy questions—"Who's the real mother?" "Which one of you is the dad?" "How did you get pregnant?" Responses:

- "We're both real mothers."
- "Neither of us is the dad—we're both mothers."
- "That's personal."
- "Interesting question. Why do you ask?"

You don't owe strangers explanations. For medical providers, provide information necessary for medical care but not intimate details of conception.

26.4 Newborn Care Basics

Basic newborn care is the same for all families regardless of structure.

Feeding: Feed on demand (8-12 times per 24 hours for newborns). Watch for hunger cues (rooting, sucking on hands, fussiness) and feed before baby is crying. Burp baby mid-feeding and after feeding by holding upright and patting or rubbing back.

Diapering: Change diapers every 2-3 hours or whenever soiled. Clean carefully, especially for babies assigned female at birth (wipe front to back). Apply diaper cream if any redness. By day 5, expect 6+ wet diapers and 3+ dirty diapers daily.

Sleep: Newborns sleep 14-17 hours per day in short stretches. Safe sleep guidelines: on back, alone in bassinet or crib, no blankets or stuffed animals, firm mattress. Room-sharing (baby in your room but separate sleep surface) reduces SIDS risk (Moon & Task Force on Sudden Infant Death Syndrome, 2016).

Bathing: Sponge baths until umbilical cord falls off (1-2 weeks), then regular baths 2-3 times per week (more frequent washing isn't necessary). Use mild soap, warm water, support baby's head, never leave baby unattended.

Cord care: Keep umbilical cord stump clean and dry. It turns black and falls off in 1-3 weeks. Call pediatrician if you see redness, drainage, or foul smell.

Soothing: Common soothing techniques include swaddling, holding and rocking, white noise, pacifier, bouncing, skin-to-skin contact, feeding. Every baby has preferences—learn what works for your specific baby.

When to call pediatrician: Fever over 100.4°F in baby under 3 months, difficulty breathing, refusing to eat for multiple feedings, fewer than 6 wet diapers daily after day 5, persistent crying you can't soothe, or anything that worries you (better to call and be reassured than miss something serious).

26.5 Partner Role Sharing

Dividing newborn care labor equitably between partners is crucial for relationship health and fairness.

If one parent is chest-feeding: The feeding parent spends significant time feeding. Balance this by having the non-feeding parent handle:

- All diaper changes
- Bringing baby to feeding parent for night feedings
- Soothing and holding between feedings
- Baths
- Laundry and household tasks
- Ordering food or cooking

If formula feeding or pumping: Split all tasks equally. Alternate who feeds for each feeding or split day into shifts (one parent handles 8am-2pm, other handles 2pm-8pm, split nights).

For single parents: All tasks fall on you. You need additional support—family, friends, hired help, or postpartum doulas. Don't try to do everything alone.

Common inequity patterns to avoid:

- Gestational parent doing everything because "you're better at it" or "baby prefers you"
- Non-gestational parent working full-time while gestational parent is home with baby and somehow still doing all night care
- Gestational parent feeling unable to ask for help
- Non-gestational partner "helping" rather than co-parenting equally

Creating equity:

- Explicitly discuss who does what tasks

- Alternate tasks rather than one person always doing specific things
- Both parents learn all aspects of baby care
- Track division of labor if needed to ensure fairness
- Adjust as needed when imbalance emerges

26.6 Circumcision Considerations

If your baby is assigned male at birth, you'll decide about circumcision—surgical removal of foreskin from penis.

Medical perspective: The American Academy of Pediatrics states that benefits of circumcision (reduced UTI risk, reduced STI risk, reduced penile cancer risk) slightly outweigh risks (bleeding, infection, surgical complications), but benefits aren't strong enough to recommend universal circumcision (American Academy of Pediatrics, 2012). It's a personal decision.

Common reasons people choose circumcision:

- Cultural or religious tradition
- Matching parent's anatomy
- Perceived cleanliness
- Belief it's "normal" in their community

Common reasons people decline circumcision:

- Belief in bodily autonomy (letting child decide later)
- Avoiding unnecessary surgery
- Growing recognition that circumcision isn't medically necessary
- Intact penis is easier to care for (no surgical recovery)

For LGBTQ+ families specifically: Some families want their son's anatomy to match that of their father or male parent if he has a penis. Others don't consider matching important. Some families explicitly choose bodily autonomy as a value, allowing their child to decide later about their own body.

Timing: If you choose circumcision, it's typically done before hospital discharge (for hospital births) or within first few weeks. Healing takes 7-10 days. If you're undecided, you can wait—circumcision can be performed later if desired, though it's more involved after newborn period.

26.7 Family and Friend Visits

Managing visitors postpartum requires setting boundaries to protect your recovery, bonding time, and sanity.

Setting boundaries:

- Limit visit length (30-60 minutes is reasonable)
- Limit number of visitors at once
- Require visitors to wash hands before holding baby
- Ask sick people to stay home
- Postpone visits if you're overwhelmed
- Have visitors help (bring food, do dishes, fold laundry) rather than creating work for you

Special considerations for LGBTQ+ families:

- If family members aren't fully supportive of your relationship or family structure, limit their visits or delay until you have energy to manage them
- Brief visitors on correct names and pronouns for transgender or non-binary parents before they arrive
- Correct people immediately if they misgender you or question your family structure
- Your partner should advocate if visitors are problematic—protect each other

Saying no: You can decline visitors. "We're not ready for visitors yet." "We need time to bond as a family." "We'll let you know when we're ready." You don't need permission to protect your postpartum period.

For unsupportive family: If biological family isn't supportive of your LGBTQ+ identity or family structure, limit their involvement or exclude them entirely. Chosen family can provide the support biological family fails to offer.

26.8 Building Your Village

New parents need support. Build your support network intentionally.

Types of support:

- **Practical help**: Meal delivery, holding baby while you nap, doing laundry, grocery shopping
- **Emotional support**: People to talk to who understand what you're going through
- **Information**: Experienced parents who can answer questions
- **Social connection**: Adult interaction so you don't feel isolated

Where to find support:

- LGBTQ+ parenting groups (in-person and online)
- New parent groups through hospitals or community centers
- Online forums and social media groups
- Friends with young children
- Postpartum doulas (paid support for postpartum period)
- Lactation consultants for feeding support
- Parenting classes
- Religious or community organizations

For LGBTQ+ parents specifically: LGBTQ+ parenting groups provide community with people who understand your specific challenges. Regular parenting groups also work if they're inclusive, but you might be the only LGBTQ+ family. Having some LGBTQ+ parent friends helps you feel less isolated.

Building chosen family: If biological family isn't supportive, intentionally build chosen family—close friends who become honorary aunts, uncles, or grandparents to your baby. Many LGBTQ+ people create family networks that provide what biological families fail to offer.

26.9 Example of Family Navigation

Consider Marcus and Tao's experience (composite): At their son's first pediatrician appointment, the intake form said "Mother" and "Father." Marcus told the receptionist "Actually, we're both fathers." She crossed out the labels and wrote "Parent 1: Marcus (he/him)" and "Parent 2: Tao (he/him)."

The pediatrician initially seemed confused—she kept glancing at Marcus's postpartum body and Tao and back to Marcus, trying to piece together how two men had a newborn. Finally she asked "I want to make sure I understand your family correctly. Who gave birth?" Marcus said "I did. I'm a transgender man." The pediatrician said "Got it, thank you for clarifying. That helps me understand your medical history."

From that point forward, the pediatrician treated them as two fathers without issue. She corrected nurses who said "mom" despite Marcus's pronouns being clearly noted in the chart. By the one-month appointment, all staff consistently used correct language.

Marcus's mother visited at two weeks postpartum and kept saying "Well, you're a mother now." Marcus corrected her: "I'm a father, not a mother." She resisted, saying "But you gave birth!" Tao stepped in: "Marcus is our son's father. Please respect that." After several corrections, she adjusted (mostly).

By three months, they had a rhythm. They'd found LGBTQ+-affirming pediatrician, completed second-parent adoption paperwork for Tao, established both fathers on all legal documents, explained their family to multiple providers, and built community with other queer parents. Their family was unconventional but thriving.

26.10 Key Newborn Navigation Points

Choose LGBTQ+-affirming pediatricians who respect your family structure, use correct pronouns, and treat all parents equally. Establish legal parentage through birth certificates and second-parent adoption where required. Explain your family to medical providers, using simple, clear scripts and setting boundaries against invasive questions.

Basic newborn care involves responsive feeding, safe sleep practices, diapering, bathing, and soothing. Divide labor equitably between partners, ensuring both parents participate fully in care. Make circumcision decisions based on your values. Manage visitors by setting boundaries protecting your recovery and family bonding.

Build support networks through LGBTQ+ parenting groups, new parent communities, and chosen family. Intentional community-building reduces isolation and provides practical help. Navigate medical systems by advocating consistently for recognition of your family structure. Your family is valid, normal, and deserving of respect from all providers and systems.

Part Six: Special Topics and Advocacy

Chapter 27.0: High Risk Pregnancy Considerations

Carmen's OB looked at her chart and said "Your Type 1 diabetes makes this a high-risk pregnancy. You'll need more frequent monitoring." Carmen felt her stomach drop. High-risk sounded scary, like something might go terribly wrong. Her wife Isabella squeezed her hand. "What does that actually mean?" Isabella asked. The OB explained: more ultrasounds, more blood tests, visits every two weeks instead of monthly, and working closely with Carmen's endocrinologist. High-risk didn't mean disaster—it meant closer monitoring to catch and prevent problems early.

High-risk pregnancies involve medical conditions or complications requiring additional monitoring and care beyond routine prenatal care. For LGBTQ+ people, accessing high-risk obstetric care involves navigating specialists who might not understand your family structure while managing genuine medical concerns. This chapter covers preexisting conditions, gestational diabetes, preeclampsia, preterm labor, multiple pregnancies, fetal complications, and accessing affirming high-risk care.

27.1 Preexisting Conditions and Pregnancy

Many people enter pregnancy with chronic health conditions requiring specialized management throughout pregnancy.

Common preexisting conditions affecting pregnancy:

Diabetes (Type 1 or Type 2): Requires tight blood sugar control throughout pregnancy to prevent complications. Uncontrolled diabetes increases risk of birth defects, preterm birth, large babies, and stillbirth. Management involves frequent blood sugar monitoring, insulin adjustments, dietary control, and regular ultrasounds to monitor fetal growth (American Diabetes Association, 2023).

Hypertension: Chronic high blood pressure increases risk of preeclampsia, placental abruption, and poor fetal growth. Medication adjustments are necessary since some blood pressure medications aren't safe in pregnancy. Close monitoring of blood pressure and fetal growth is required.

Thyroid disorders: Both hypothyroidism and hyperthyroidism affect pregnancy. Hypothyroidism requires increased thyroid hormone replacement during pregnancy. Hyperthyroidism might require medication adjustment. Uncontrolled thyroid disorders increase miscarriage risk and affect fetal development.

Autoimmune conditions: Lupus, rheumatoid arthritis, and other autoimmune diseases require specialized care. Some conditions improve during pregnancy, others worsen. Medications often need adjustment since many immunosuppressants aren't safe in pregnancy.

Cardiac conditions: Heart disease complicates pregnancy because pregnancy increases cardiac workload. Depending on condition severity, some people are advised against pregnancy due to maternal health risks.

Mental health conditions: Depression, anxiety, bipolar disorder, and other mental health conditions require continued treatment during pregnancy. Many psychiatric medications are safe in pregnancy, though some require switching to safer alternatives.

For transgender men: If you have preexisting conditions from testosterone use (polycythemia, lipid changes, etc.), these typically resolve after stopping testosterone. Discuss any ongoing health concerns with your provider.

27.2 Gestational Diabetes

Gestational diabetes develops during pregnancy in people who didn't previously have diabetes, affecting about 6-9% of pregnancies (American College of Obstetricians and Gynecologists, 2022).

What causes gestational diabetes: Pregnancy hormones make your body resistant to insulin. Most people's pancreas compensates by making more insulin, but some can't produce enough, causing high blood sugar.

Screening: All pregnant people are screened for gestational diabetes between 24-28 weeks with a glucose tolerance test. You drink a sugary solution and have blood drawn one or three hours later to measure blood sugar response.

Management if diagnosed:

- Blood sugar monitoring four times daily (fasting and after meals)
- Dietary changes (controlled carbohydrates, balanced meals)
- Regular exercise
- Insulin or metformin if diet and exercise don't control blood sugar
- More frequent prenatal visits and ultrasounds
- Fetal monitoring to check baby's size and wellbeing

Complications if uncontrolled: Large babies (making vaginal delivery difficult), preterm birth, low blood sugar in baby after birth, increased cesarean risk, future diabetes risk for both parent and baby.

After birth: Gestational diabetes typically resolves immediately after delivery, but having it increases your risk of developing Type 2 diabetes later. Postpartum glucose testing at 6-12 weeks checks whether diabetes persists.

27.3 Preeclampsia

Preeclampsia is a serious pregnancy complication involving high blood pressure and often protein in urine, affecting 5-8% of pregnancies (American College of Obstetricians and Gynecologists, 2020).

Signs and symptoms:

- High blood pressure (140/90 or higher)
- Protein in urine
- Severe headaches
- Vision changes (blurriness, seeing spots)
- Upper abdominal pain
- Sudden severe swelling of hands and face
- Decreased urine output

Risk factors: First pregnancy, pregnancy over age 35, obesity, chronic hypertension, diabetes, kidney disease, autoimmune conditions, carrying multiples, history of preeclampsia in previous pregnancy.

Why it's dangerous: Preeclampsia restricts blood flow to placenta, causing poor fetal growth. Severe preeclampsia can progress to eclampsia (seizures), stroke, organ damage, or HELLP syndrome (a life-threatening complication affecting liver and blood clotting).

Management:

- Close monitoring of blood pressure and symptoms
- Regular urine protein testing
- Blood tests monitoring liver and kidney function
- Ultrasounds checking fetal growth
- Possible bed rest or reduced activity
- Medications to lower blood pressure
- Hospitalization if severe
- Early delivery if condition worsens (often between 34-37 weeks)

Cure: The only cure for preeclampsia is delivery. After birth, blood pressure typically returns to normal, though postpartum preeclampsia can develop even after delivery.

27.4 Preterm Labor

Preterm labor—labor beginning before 37 weeks—occurs in about 10% of pregnancies and is a leading cause of infant complications (March of Dimes, 2023).

Warning signs:

- Regular contractions (more than four per hour)
- Pelvic pressure or cramping
- Low backache that comes and goes
- Watery fluid leaking from vagina
- Change in vaginal discharge (bloody, mucus-like)

Risk factors: Previous preterm birth, carrying multiples, uterine or cervical abnormalities, infections, chronic stress, smoking, inadequate prenatal care, certain medical conditions.

What happens if preterm labor starts: Your provider checks cervical dilation and fetal wellbeing. If you're in active preterm labor before 34 weeks, interventions might include:

- Tocolytic medications to stop contractions temporarily
- Corticosteroids to speed fetal lung development
- Magnesium sulfate to protect baby's brain
- Antibiotics if infection suspected
- Hospital bed rest and monitoring
- Transfer to hospital with NICU if birth seems imminent

Outcomes: Babies born prematurely face risks depending on gestational age. Babies born after 34 weeks typically do well with minimal complications. Earlier births (28-33 weeks) require NICU care but most survive and develop normally. Very premature births (before 28 weeks) involve significant complications and long NICU stays.

27.5 Multiple Pregnancy

Carrying twins, triplets, or more automatically classifies pregnancy as high-risk, requiring specialized monitoring throughout.

Complications with multiples:

- Increased risk of preterm birth (average twin delivery: 35-36 weeks)
- Higher rates of gestational diabetes
- Increased preeclampsia risk
- Greater likelihood of cesarean delivery
- More severe pregnancy symptoms
- Twin-to-twin transfusion syndrome (in identical twins sharing placenta)
- Growth restriction if babies are sharing resources

Monitoring: Ultrasounds every 4-6 weeks to check fetal growth, amniotic fluid, and placental function. More frequent visits to monitor for preeclampsia and preterm labor.

Delivery timing: Most twin pregnancies deliver between 36-38 weeks. Many providers recommend delivery by 38 weeks even if labor hasn't started, to reduce stillbirth risk.

For LGBTQ+ families: Some fertility treatments (particularly IVF) increase multiple pregnancy risk. If carrying multiples from fertility treatment, you'll need high-risk obstetric care from providers who understand assisted reproduction and LGBTQ+ family building.

27.6 Fetal Complications

Sometimes complications arise with the baby rather than the pregnant person.

Growth restriction: Baby measuring small for gestational age might indicate placental insufficiency, chromosomal abnormalities, or maternal health conditions. Requires frequent ultrasounds and sometimes early delivery if baby isn't thriving.

Fetal anomalies: Structural abnormalities detected on ultrasound might require pediatric surgery after birth, specialized delivery at tertiary care center, or in severe cases, decisions about pregnancy continuation.

Placental problems: Placenta previa (placenta covering cervix) requires cesarean delivery and careful monitoring for bleeding. Placental abruption (placenta separating from uterus prematurely) is an emergency requiring immediate delivery.

Oligohydramnios or polyhydramnios: Too little or too much amniotic fluid can indicate fetal problems, requiring investigation and monitoring.

Rh incompatibility: If you're Rh-negative and baby is Rh-positive, your body might produce antibodies against baby's blood. Prevented with RhoGAM injections during pregnancy and after birth.

When fetal complications are diagnosed: You'll be referred to maternal-fetal medicine specialists and possibly pediatric specialists. Decisions about monitoring, early delivery, and postnatal care depend on specific complications.

27.7 Accessing High Risk Care

High-risk obstetric care involves maternal-fetal medicine (MFM) specialists—OBs with additional training in complicated pregnancies.

What MFM care involves:

- Detailed ultrasounds evaluating fetal anatomy and growth
- Non-stress tests monitoring fetal heart rate

- Biophysical profiles combining ultrasound and heart rate monitoring
- Consultation on pregnancy management and delivery timing
- Coordination with other specialists (endocrinologists, cardiologists, etc.)
- More frequent appointments than routine prenatal care

Finding LGBTQ+ affirming MFM care: High-risk care requires even more medical interactions than routine pregnancy, making affirming care even more important. Look for:

- MFM practices advertising LGBTQ+ competency
- Recommendations from LGBTQ+ parents or organizations
- Academic medical centers (often more inclusive than private practices)
- Practices with experience in gestational surrogacy (indicates they work with diverse family structures)

Advocating in high-risk care settings: With multiple specialists involved, you'll need to repeatedly clarify your family structure, correct pronouns, and ensure all providers recognize both parents. Bring your partner to all appointments and insist they're included in conversations and decision-making.

For transgender men: MFM specialists might have never cared for pregnant transgender men before. Be prepared to educate. Bring written information about transgender pregnancy if needed. Don't accept disrespectful care—advocate for yourself or switch providers if necessary.

27.8 Real High Risk Experience

Consider Isabella and Carmen's journey (composite): Carmen's Type 1 diabetes meant high-risk care from the start. She met with an MFM specialist at 12 weeks who explained the monitoring plan: ultrasounds every 4 weeks starting at 16 weeks, non-stress tests twice weekly starting at 32 weeks, frequent visits with her OB and endocrinologist.

The MFM specialist initially only addressed Carmen, ignoring Isabella entirely. Isabella interrupted: "I'm Carmen's wife and this baby's other mother. I need to hear all of this too." The specialist apologized and started directing information to both of them.

Carmen's blood sugars stayed well-controlled throughout pregnancy with frequent insulin adjustments. Ultrasounds showed baby growing normally. At 36 weeks, the MFM recommended induction at 38 weeks to reduce stillbirth risk associated with diabetes.

Isabella and Carmen delivered at 38 weeks exactly. Their daughter was healthy, though she spent 6 hours in the nursery for blood sugar monitoring (common with diabetic pregnancies). By 12 hours old, her blood sugars were stable and she came to their room.

Looking back, Carmen was grateful for high-risk care—the close monitoring gave her confidence that problems would be caught early. Yes, it meant more appointments and more anxiety, but it meant their daughter was born healthy despite the complications.

27.9 Key High Risk Points

High-risk pregnancies involve preexisting medical conditions or pregnancy complications requiring specialized monitoring. Common conditions include diabetes, hypertension, thyroid disorders, autoimmune diseases, and cardiac problems. Gestational diabetes affects 6-9% of pregnancies and requires blood sugar monitoring, dietary changes, and sometimes medication.

Preeclampsia is a dangerous complication involving high blood pressure requiring close monitoring and sometimes early delivery. Preterm labor before 37 weeks affects 10% of pregnancies and requires interventions to delay delivery and support fetal development. Multiple pregnancies automatically require high-risk care due to increased complication rates.

Fetal complications like growth restriction or anomalies require maternal-fetal medicine consultation. Accessing affirming high-risk care involves finding LGBTQ+ competent MFM specialists and advocating throughout care. High-risk designation doesn't mean disaster—it means closer monitoring to optimize outcomes for both parent and baby.

Chapter 28.0: Pregnancy Loss and Grief

Maya held the ultrasound wand against her belly at 11 weeks, waiting to see the heartbeat. The technician was quiet for too long. Then: "I'm so sorry. There's no heartbeat. Your baby stopped developing around 8 weeks." The world tilted. Jordan, Maya's partner, started crying. Maya felt numb. They'd already told their families, picked out names, imagined their future. Now what? The pregnancy was over, but their baby was still inside Maya's body. They had to decide how to end it—medication, surgery, or waiting for miscarriage to start naturally. Nothing about this was fair or okay.

Pregnancy loss is devastating and far more common than most people realize—about 10-20% of known pregnancies end in miscarriage, with even higher rates for very early losses (American College of Obstetricians and Gynecologists, 2021). This chapter covers miscarriage, stillbirth, neonatal loss, medical management of loss, grief in LGBTQ+ families, partner grief, trying again, and memorial practices.

28.1 Early Miscarriage

Miscarriage—pregnancy loss before 20 weeks—occurs in 10-20% of known pregnancies, with most losses in the first trimester.

Common causes:

- Chromosomal abnormalities in embryo or fetus (most common cause)
- Uterine abnormalities
- Hormonal problems
- Infection
- Chronic health conditions
- Unknown (many miscarriages have no identifiable cause)

Important: Miscarriage is almost never caused by anything the pregnant person did. Exercise, sex, stress, lifting, or working don't cause miscarriage. Most losses result from random genetic errors, not from any action or inaction.

Signs of miscarriage:

- Bleeding (light spotting to heavy bleeding)
- Cramping
- Loss of pregnancy symptoms
- Tissue or clot passage

Types of early loss:

Missed miscarriage: Embryo stops developing but body doesn't recognize loss immediately. Often discovered at routine ultrasound showing no heartbeat.

Incomplete miscarriage: Miscarriage begins but some tissue remains in uterus.

Complete miscarriage: All pregnancy tissue passes naturally.

Blighted ovum: Gestational sac forms but embryo never develops inside it.

Medical management options: When miscarriage is diagnosed but hasn't completed naturally, three options exist:

- Expectant management (waiting for natural miscarriage)
- Medication (misoprostol to cause cramping and bleeding to expel tissue)
- D&C (dilation and curettage—surgical removal of tissue under anesthesia)

Each option has pros and cons regarding timing, pain, bleeding, and emotional impact.

28.2 Late Miscarriage

Miscarriage between 13-20 weeks is less common but more physically and emotionally difficult than early loss.

Differences from early loss: By second trimester, you're visibly pregnant, have felt movement, and had detailed ultrasounds. Loss at this stage feels more like losing a baby than an abstract pregnancy.

Physical experience: Second-trimester loss often involves labor—contractions, cervical dilation, and delivery of a recognizable fetus. This is traumatic for many people.

Medical management: D&E (dilation and evacuation) procedure is typically offered as alternative to labor. This involves cervical dilation over 1-2 days followed by surgical removal of pregnancy tissue under anesthesia.

Decision-making: Choosing between D&E and labor induction is deeply personal. Some people want to avoid labor and delivery. Others want to see and hold their baby. Neither choice is wrong.

Seeing and holding baby: Hospitals typically offer the option to see, hold, and photograph babies lost after about 16 weeks. Some people find this healing and important for their grief process. Others don't want to. Both are valid.

28.3 Stillbirth

Stillbirth—fetal death after 20 weeks—occurs in about 1 in 160 pregnancies (American College of Obstetricians and Gynecologists, 2021).

Common causes:

- Placental problems (abruption, insufficiency)
- Birth defects
- Infection
- Umbilical cord accidents
- Maternal health conditions
- Unknown (nearly half of stillbirths have no identifiable cause)

How stillbirth is discovered: Sometimes detected at routine appointments when provider can't find heartbeat. Sometimes pregnant person notices decreased fetal movement and comes in for evaluation.

Delivery after stillbirth: Most people deliver vaginally after stillbirth unless there's medical reason for cesarean. Labor is typically induced within a day or two of diagnosis. Some people want immediate induction; others need time to process before delivery.

Physical recovery: After stillbirth, your body still goes through postpartum changes—milk comes in, bleeding lasts for weeks, hormones shift dramatically. These physical reminders of pregnancy without a living baby are cruel.

Seeing baby: Hospitals strongly encourage seeing and holding stillborn babies, taking photos, collecting footprints and handprints, and keeping mementos. Research shows this helps with grief and doesn't increase psychological harm (Cassidy, 2018).

Autopsy and testing: Trying to determine why stillbirth occurred involves autopsy, placental examination, and genetic testing. Results might provide answers or might find nothing—both outcomes are hard.

28.4 Neonatal Loss

Neonatal loss—baby's death within first 28 days of life—occurs after premature birth, birth complications, or congenital abnormalities incompatible with life.

Differences from stillbirth: You've met your baby, held them alive, heard them cry or breathe. Losing them after birth involves saying goodbye to a person you knew, not just a pregnancy you carried.

NICU loss: Many neonatal deaths occur in NICU after days or weeks of treatment. You bond with your baby, hope for improvement, then lose them. This extended grief and hope-fear cycle is exhausting.

Decision-making about care: Sometimes neonatal loss involves decisions about ending life support or withdrawing aggressive treatment. These are agonizing decisions with no right answer.

Time with baby after death: Hospitals typically allow extended time with baby after death—hours or even days. You can hold them, take photos, have family meet them, and say goodbye on your timeline.

Physical and emotional recovery: After neonatal loss, your body recovered from birth but you have no baby. Milk production, postpartum bleeding, and hormonal changes continue while you grieve.

28.5 Medical Management Details

Understanding medical procedures and physical experiences after loss helps you make informed decisions.

Miscarriage management:

Expectant management: Waiting for natural miscarriage. Might take days or weeks. Involves unpredictable timing and heavy bleeding. Some people prefer this to avoid medications or procedures.

Medication (misoprostol): Causes cramping and bleeding to expel pregnancy tissue. Given as vaginal tablets or oral pills. Cramping can be severe. Bleeding lasts for days to weeks. Success rate about 85%. If unsuccessful, D&C is needed.

D&C procedure: Performed in operating room under anesthesia. Cervix is dilated and tissue removed with suction and scraping. Takes 15-20 minutes. Recovery is quick—bleeding for 1-2 weeks, return to normal activities within days. Risks include infection, uterine perforation (rare), and Asherman's syndrome (rare scarring).

After second-trimester loss or stillbirth:

Labor induction: Medications (misoprostol and/or oxytocin) start labor and contractions. Epidural is available for pain management. Labor typically lasts 12-24 hours. After delivery, placenta is delivered and provider checks that uterus is empty.

D&E procedure: Cervical dilation over 1-2 days using dilators, then surgical removal of pregnancy tissue under anesthesia. Avoids labor and delivery but requires two-day process.

Physical recovery timeline: Regardless of loss type, physical recovery takes weeks. Bleeding lasts 2-6 weeks. Hormones shift dramatically. Milk might come in after second-trimester or later loss. Next period typically returns in 4-6 weeks.

28.6 Grief in LGBTQ+ Families

LGBTQ+ families face unique challenges with pregnancy loss due to lack of recognition and additional losses.

Lack of recognition: Society often minimizes pregnancy loss. For LGBTQ+ families, loss might be further minimized because your family was already considered "less legitimate." People might not recognize how devastating this loss is.

Financial loss: If you used fertility treatments, donors, or surrogacy, pregnancy loss involves massive financial loss on top of emotional loss. Money invested in trying to build your family is gone with nothing to show for it.

Timeline loss: Pregnancy loss might mean months or years before trying again due to time needed to save money, find new donors, or redo fertility treatments. This extended timeline before another attempt amplifies grief.

For transgender men: Pregnancy loss involves complicated grief—losing a pregnancy you endured severe dysphoria to carry, with nothing to show for that sacrifice. The dysphoria wasn't worth it because there's no baby.

Disenfranchised grief: Society doesn't always recognize or validate your grief because your family structure is already questioned. This makes processing grief harder.

28.7 Partner Grief Experiences

Non-gestational partners grieve pregnancy loss too, though their grief is often invisible or minimized.

Partner's grief: You lost this baby too. You dreamed of parenthood, picked names, imagined your future, and lost all of it. Your grief is real and valid.

Watching your partner suffer: Non-gestational partners watch their partners go through physical trauma of miscarriage or stillbirth while feeling helpless. You can't fix this or make it better. That helplessness is agonizing.

Lack of recognition: Medical systems focus on the pregnant person. Family and friends ask how your partner is doing, not how you're doing. Your grief becomes invisible.

Supporting while grieving: Non-gestational partners often feel they need to be strong for their grieving partner while suppressing their own grief. This is unsustainable. You need support too.

Different grief timelines: Partners often grieve differently and on different timelines. One might be ready to try again before the other. This creates relationship strain. Communication and patience are essential.

28.8 Trying Again

Deciding whether and when to try again after pregnancy loss is deeply personal.

Physical readiness: Medically, you can typically try again after one normal menstrual cycle following miscarriage. After stillbirth or second-trimester loss, waiting 3-6 months is sometimes recommended for physical recovery, though evidence doesn't show increased risk with earlier attempts (Wong et al., 2016).

Emotional readiness: Emotional readiness takes longer than physical readiness for most people. You might need months to grieve, process trauma, and feel ready to risk this pain again. Don't rush based on others' timelines.

Fear in subsequent pregnancy: Pregnancy after loss involves intense anxiety. Every twinge causes panic. You might not feel excited or connected to subsequent pregnancies until much later. This is normal.

Testing and interventions: After multiple losses (typically 2-3 consecutive losses), providers run tests looking for causes—chromosomal testing, hormone testing, uterine imaging, blood clotting disorders. Sometimes cause is found and addressed. Often nothing is found and you just try again.

For LGBTQ+ families: Trying again might require repeating expensive fertility treatments, finding new donors, or returning to surrogacy agencies. The financial and logistical barriers to trying again are significant beyond emotional barriers.

28.9 Memorial and Healing Practices

Rituals and practices honoring lost pregnancies help many people process grief.

Memorial practices:

- Naming your baby (even early losses)
- Planting a tree or garden
- Creating memory box with ultrasound photos, hospital bands, footprints
- Jewelry containing baby's birthstone or ashes
- Tattoos commemorating loss
- Charitable donations in baby's name
- Funeral or memorial service (particularly after stillbirth or neonatal loss)

Burial and cremation: After stillbirth or neonatal loss, you can arrange burial or cremation for your baby. Funeral homes often provide reduced rates or free services for infant loss. Some hospitals provide free cremation.

Support groups: Pregnancy loss support groups (in-person or online) connect you with others who understand this specific grief.

Sharing experiences and supporting others who understand is healing for many people.

Therapy: Grief therapy or trauma therapy helps process loss, manage anxiety in subsequent pregnancies, and work through complicated feelings. Not everyone needs therapy after loss, but it's available if you do.

LGBTQ+ specific support: Some pregnancy loss support groups are LGBTQ+ specific, recognizing the particular challenges of loss in our community. These spaces allow processing grief without having to explain your family structure.

28.10 Composite Loss Journey

Consider Chen and Michael's experience (composite): Chen miscarried at 10 weeks. They'd conceived using IVF after two failed IUI cycles, investing $18,000 and 18 months of effort. When ultrasound showed no heartbeat, Chen felt defeated. Michael felt guilty that his grief was about money and time when Chen lost an actual pregnancy from his body.

Chen chose medication management. The cramping was excruciating, worse than anything he expected. Michael held him while he cried and bled and passed tissue. The physical ordeal lasted 12 hours. The emotional aftermath lasted months.

They joined a pregnancy loss support group where Michael finally heard other partners express similar guilt about grieving differently than gestational parents. Chen found therapy to process the trauma of miscarriage and the dysphoria that intensified with pregnancy loss.

Six months later, they tried IVF again. Chen was pregnant again at 11 weeks when his first loss would have been due. He couldn't feel excited—just terrified of losing this pregnancy too. Every ultrasound brought panic until they heard a heartbeat.

At 20 weeks, they finally exhaled slightly. By 30 weeks, they started believing they'd actually have a baby. At 39 weeks, their daughter was born healthy. The grief from miscarriage never disappeared, but it existed alongside joy about their daughter. Both feelings were real and valid simultaneously.

28.11 Core Loss Principles

Pregnancy loss affects 10-20% of known pregnancies, occurring most commonly in first trimester but also happening in second trimester (late miscarriage), after 20 weeks (stillbirth), or after birth (neonatal loss). Causes include chromosomal abnormalities, placental problems, maternal health conditions, and often no identifiable cause. Miscarriage management options include expectant management, medication, or D&C procedures.

LGBTQ+ families face compounded grief due to lack of recognition, financial losses from fertility treatment, and extended timelines before trying again. Non-gestational partners grieve too but often face invisible grief and pressure to support without acknowledging their own loss. Deciding when to try again involves both physical and emotional readiness, with subsequent pregnancies typically filled with anxiety.

Memorial practices like naming babies, creating memory boxes, planting trees, or holding services help many people process grief. Support groups, therapy, and time facilitate healing, though grief from pregnancy loss doesn't disappear completely—it transforms over time. Your loss is real, your grief is valid, and you deserve support regardless of how early the loss occurred or your family structure.

Chapter 29.0: Legal Rights and Documentation

Aisha and Layla's daughter was born on a Tuesday. By Wednesday, they were filling out birth certificate paperwork. The form said "Mother" and "Father." Aisha told the hospital registrar "We're both mothers." The registrar looked confused, then said "Let me check with my supervisor." Thirty minutes later she returned: "Sorry, our state doesn't allow two mothers on birth certificates. One of you has to be listed as father." Aisha and Layla were furious. This was 2023, same-sex marriage had been legal for eight years, and their state still didn't recognize their family. They refused to fill out the form incorrectly and hired an attorney to fix it.

Legal recognition of LGBTQ+ families varies dramatically by location, with some states fully recognizing same-sex parents automatically and others requiring lengthy legal processes to establish both parents' rights. This chapter covers birth certificate completion, second-parent adoption, name and gender marker changes, travel with babies, healthcare decision-making, estate planning, discrimination recourse, and legal resources.

29.1 Birth Certificate Completion

Birth certificates establish legal parentage and are required for numerous purposes—enrolling in school, obtaining passports, accessing healthcare, proving identity.

How birth certificates work: When a baby is born, hospital staff complete vital statistics paperwork including both parents' information. This information goes to the state vital records office, which issues the official birth certificate.

For married same-sex couples: In 2017, the Supreme Court case *Pavan v. Smith* established that states must list both spouses on birth certificates regardless of sex (Obergefell v. Hodges, 2015; Pavan v. Smith, 2017). However, implementation varies. Some states comply fully. Others resist.

What to do at hospital:

- Fill out forms with both parents' names
- List the non-gestational parent in the appropriate parent field (not as "father" if they're not male)
- If hospital staff resist, cite *Pavan v. Smith*
- Document any resistance for potential legal action
- Don't accept incorrect forms to avoid conflict

For unmarried same-sex couples: Most states require second-parent adoption for the non-biological parent, even in long-term committed relationships. The initial birth certificate lists only the gestational parent.

For transgender men: Some states allow you to be listed as "father" on your child's birth certificate. Others list you as "mother" despite being male. This varies by state and sometimes by county. If misgendered on the birth certificate, you can petition courts to correct it.

For gender markers: Most birth certificates include baby's sex assigned at birth. Some states now offer non-binary options (X instead of M or F) if requested. This is rare but growing.

Correcting errors: If the birth certificate is issued incorrectly, you can file corrections through the state vital records office or through courts. Don't accept incorrect birth certificates—they'll cause problems for years.

29.2 Second Parent Adoption Process

Second-parent adoption legally establishes the non-biological parent's legal relationship to their child. This is required in many states for unmarried couples and sometimes even for married couples.

Why it's necessary: Without legal parentage, the non-biological parent has no automatic rights to make medical decisions, no custody rights if the relationship ends, and no rights if the biological parent dies. Second-parent adoption protects your family legally.

The process:

Step 1: File petition: Work with an LGBTQ+ family law attorney to file a second-parent adoption petition with your local court. This includes paperwork about both parents, the child, and your relationship.

Step 2: Home study (if required): Some states require home studies evaluating your home environment and parenting capacity. This feels invasive—a social worker visits your home, interviews you, and writes a report. Other states waive home studies for second-parent adoptions.

Step 3: Background checks: Most jurisdictions require criminal background checks and child abuse clearances.

Step 4: Hearing: A court hearing finalizes the adoption. This is typically brief and procedural—the judge asks a few questions and signs the order establishing legal parentage.

Step 5: Amended birth certificate: After adoption is finalized, you receive an amended birth certificate listing both parents.

Timeline: Second-parent adoption typically takes 3-6 months from filing to finalization, depending on your state's requirements and court schedules.

Cost: Attorney fees range from $1,500-$5,000. Court filing fees add several hundred dollars. Home study fees (if required) add $1,000-$3,000.

For gay male couples using surrogacy: The process is similar but often more complicated because neither parent gave birth. Both parents might need to adopt, or you might establish parentage through pre-birth orders (available in some states).

29.3 Name and Gender Changes

Transgender parents might need to change their name or gender marker on legal documents related to their children.

Changing your own documents: If you haven't legally changed your name or gender marker, having children might motivate you to do so. Processes vary by state but typically involve:

- Filing petition with court
- Publishing notice in newspaper (in some states)
- Attending court hearing
- Obtaining court order
- Updating driver's license, passport, Social Security records
- Timeline: 2-6 months

Birth certificates listing wrong gender: If your child's birth certificate lists you with wrong gender (e.g., listing you as "mother" when you're a man), you can petition the court to correct it. This requires your updated identity documents and sometimes a separate court order.

Medical records: Hospitals and clinics often misgender transgender parents in medical records. You can request corrections, though this is often challenging. Document all misgendering for potential discrimination complaints.

School and childcare: When enrolling children in school or childcare, you'll provide identification and birth certificates. If documents don't match your current name or gender, this creates complications. Having updated documents prevents problems.

29.4 Interstate and International Travel

Traveling with babies when you're an LGBTQ+ family requires preparation.

Domestic travel: Within the U.S., traveling is generally straightforward if you have ID showing both parents. For air travel, TSA doesn't require proof of parentage. Potential issues arise if traveling alone with baby and names don't match—carry the birth certificate showing you're the parent.

Interstate complications: If you established legal parentage in one state and travel to or move to a less LGBTQ+-friendly state, your legal parentage should still be recognized under full faith and credit laws. However, you might encounter resistance.

International travel: More complicated. You'll need:

Passport for baby: Requires both parents' presence at passport office or notarized permission from absent parent. Both parents must sign application. Passport lists baby's name and sex but not parents' names.

Documentation proving parentage: Birth certificate or adoption decree. Some countries require additional documentation proving both parents' legal relationship to child.

Marriage certificate: If married, bring certified marriage certificate. Some countries don't recognize same-sex marriages and might question your family structure.

Letter of consent: If one parent is traveling internationally with baby without the other parent, carry a notarized letter from the absent parent consenting to travel.

Research destination laws: Some countries criminalize homosexuality or don't recognize same-sex relationships. Research whether your destination is safe for LGBTQ+ families before traveling.

29.5 Healthcare Decision Making Authority

Legal parentage determines who can make medical decisions for your child.

If you have legal parentage: You have full authority to consent to medical treatment, make healthcare decisions, and access medical records. Providers must recognize your authority.

If you don't have legal parentage: You have NO legal authority, even if you're the non-biological parent in a long-term relationship. The biological parent must consent to all treatment. You can't access medical records or make decisions even in emergencies.

Why this matters: If the biological parent is unavailable or incapacitated, the non-legal parent has no rights to make emergency medical decisions for their own child. This is dangerous.

Protections without legal parentage: Some states allow parents to designate medical decision-makers through forms. These are weaker than legal parentage but better than nothing. However, providers might not honor them in emergencies.

The solution: Establish legal parentage through second-parent adoption or proper birth certificate completion. This is the only way to ensure both parents have full decision-making authority.

29.6 Estate Planning

All new parents need estate planning, but LGBTQ+ families have additional considerations.

Essential documents:

Wills: Designate who gets custody of your children if both parents die. Without wills, courts decide custody—potentially giving your children to biological family members hostile to LGBTQ+ people.

Guardianship designations: Name who will raise your children if you can't. Choose guardians who will honor your values and tell your children positive things about you.

Life insurance: Provides financial support if a parent dies. Particularly important if one parent stays home or reduces work.

Healthcare proxies: Allow designated person to make medical decisions for you if you're incapacitated. Essential for protecting LGBTQ+ relationships.

Power of attorney: Allows designated person to handle financial and legal matters if you're incapacitated.

Trusts (if assets warrant): Protect assets for children and allow more control over inheritance distribution than wills alone.

Special LGBTQ+ considerations: Name specific guardians, not "family." Specify that you want LGBTQ+-affirming guardians. Consider whether biological family members would honor your wishes about your children's upbringing.

Updating documents: Update estate planning documents after any major life change—marriage, divorce, additional children, moving states.

Finding attorneys: Work with attorneys experienced in LGBTQ+ estate planning. They understand the specific vulnerabilities LGBTQ+ families face.

29.7 Discrimination and Legal Recourse

If you experience discrimination based on sexual orientation, gender identity, or family structure, legal recourse exists.

Types of discrimination:

- Healthcare providers refusing care based on sexual orientation or gender identity
- Hospitals refusing to list both parents on birth certificates
- State agencies refusing to process adoption or parentage paperwork correctly
- Schools or childcare refusing enrollment
- Housing discrimination
- Employment discrimination

Federal protections: Under *Bostock v. Clayton County* (2020), employment discrimination based on sexual orientation or gender identity violates Title VII. Healthcare discrimination might violate the Affordable Care Act. Protections continue evolving.

State protections: About 23 states explicitly prohibit discrimination based on sexual orientation and gender identity in employment, housing, and public accommodations. Other states have no protections.

Filing complaints:

Healthcare discrimination: File complaints with the U.S. Department of Health and Human Services Office for Civil Rights, state health departments, and professional licensing boards.

Vital records discrimination: Contact the state vital records office, the state attorney general's office, and national LGBTQ+ legal organizations like Lambda Legal or National Center for Lesbian Rights.

Employment discrimination: File with the Equal Employment Opportunity Commission and state civil rights agencies.

Housing discrimination: File with the U.S. Department of Housing and Urban Development and state fair housing agencies.

Legal advocacy organizations: National organizations providing free or low-cost legal help to LGBTQ+ people include Lambda Legal, ACLU LGBT Project, National Center for Lesbian Rights, and Transgender Law Center. Contact them for assistance with discrimination.

29.8 Example Legal Journey

Consider Marcus and David's experience (composite): They had twin daughters via surrogacy in California. California law allowed pre-birth orders establishing both fathers' legal parentage before birth. Their daughters' birth certificates listed both fathers correctly.

A year later, they moved to Texas for David's job. When enrolling the twins in childcare, staff questioned whether Marcus was really a parent since he wasn't the biological father. Marcus showed the birth certificate listing both fathers. Staff accepted it but made comments questioning their family.

When one twin needed emergency surgery, hospital staff initially refused to let Marcus sign consent forms because he "wasn't the real father." Marcus pulled out the birth certificate again and told the charge nurse "I am a legal parent. I have full decision-making authority. This is discrimination if you refuse to let me consent to treatment for my daughter." The nurse backed down and accepted his consent.

Marcus and David consulted with an LGBTQ+ attorney about whether they needed to do anything to protect their legal status in Texas. The attorney assured them their California parentage was valid nationwide but recommended updating estate planning documents to explicitly protect against Texas's less-friendly legal climate.

They also pre-enrolled in a second-parent adoption process as backup protection, though technically unnecessary given their pre-birth order. The legal complexity and vulnerability of their family in less-friendly states was exhausting, but they took every protective step possible.

29.9 Essential Legal Knowledge

Birth certificates establish legal parentage, with some states fully recognizing same-sex parents and others resisting despite Supreme Court precedent. Second-parent adoption is often necessary to legally protect non-biological parents' rights, involving a 3-6 month legal process including petitions, possible home studies, and court hearings.

Transgender parents might need to correct birth certificates listing wrong gender. Interstate and international travel requires proper documentation including passports, birth certificates, and sometimes consent letters. Legal parentage determines healthcare decision-making authority—without it, non-biological parents have no legal rights even in emergencies.

Estate planning protects LGBTQ+ families by designating guardians, creating wills, and establishing healthcare proxies. Discrimination based on sexual orientation or gender identity is illegal under federal law in employment and healthcare, with additional state protections varying. Legal advocacy organizations provide free support for discrimination cases. Protecting your family legally requires proactive documentation and understanding of your rights.

Chapter 30.0: Advocacy and Creating Change

Riley walked into the hospital for their 36-week ultrasound and saw the intake forms waiting at reception. "Mother's Name" and "Father's Name" stared back at them. Again. They'd corrected these forms at every appointment for nine months. Each time, staff promised to fix the forms. Each time, nothing changed. Riley was exhausted from advocating, from educating, from fighting just to have their family recognized. But they also knew: if they didn't push for change, the next LGBTQ+ family using this hospital would face the same erasure. So Riley asked to speak to the patient advocate. Again.

Advocacy means standing up for yourself and others, pushing systems to change, and making the world safer for LGBTQ+ families. Individual advocacy protects your specific family. Systemic advocacy creates lasting change benefiting all LGBTQ+ families who come after you. This chapter covers self-advocacy throughout your journey, filing discrimination complaints, working with patient advocates, educating providers, sharing your story, supporting policy change, and building LGBTQ+ parent community.

30.1 Self Advocacy Throughout Pregnancy

Self-advocacy means clearly communicating your needs, correcting mistakes, and insisting on respectful treatment.

When to self-advocate: Every time someone misgenders you, ignores your partner, uses wrong language, or treats your family as less legitimate than heterosexual/cisgender families.

How to self-advocate effectively:

Be direct and specific: Don't hint or hope providers will figure it out. State clearly: "My pronouns are he/him. Please use them consistently." "We're both mothers. Don't call me 'mom' and her 'partner.'" "I need you to include my wife in all medical discussions."

Correct immediately: When providers make mistakes, correct them right away. "Actually, I'm the father, not the mother." "Her name is Carmen, not Karen—please check your notes." Immediate correction prevents mistakes from becoming patterns.

Escalate when necessary: If frontline staff won't make changes, ask for supervisors. If supervisors don't help, contact patient advocates or administrators. Keep escalating until someone with authority responds.

Document everything: Write down dates, names of staff, what was said, and what actions you requested. Documentation is essential if you need to file formal complaints.

Bring support: Your partner can advocate with you. Having two people stating the same concern carries more weight than one.

Know your rights: Understanding legal protections helps you advocate effectively. Cite specific laws or policies when relevant: "Under this hospital's non-discrimination policy, you must use my correct name and pronouns."

Pick your battles: You can't fight every microaggression or you'll be exhausted. Focus advocacy on issues affecting your care quality or family recognition. Let minor things go sometimes for your own sanity.

30.2 Filing Discrimination Complaints

When self-advocacy doesn't work, formal complaints create accountability.

When to file complaints:

- Provider refuses care based on sexual orientation or gender identity
- Repeated misgendering despite corrections
- Exclusion of non-gestational parent from care
- Refusal to list both parents on birth certificates or medical records
- Harassment or hostile treatment
- Denial of hospital visitation for partners
- Any treatment you wouldn't receive if you were heterosexual or cisgender

Where to file:

Hospital patient relations or patient advocate office: Start here for hospital-based problems. Most hospitals have formal complaint processes. File complaints in writing detailing specific incidents, dates, staff involved, and harm caused.

State medical licensing boards: For individual providers engaging in discrimination or unprofessional conduct. Complaints can result in investigations and disciplinary action.

U.S. Department of Health and Human Services Office for Civil Rights: For healthcare discrimination based on sex, including sexual orientation and gender identity under *Bostock* precedent. File online at hhs.gov/ocr.

State civil rights agencies: Many states have civil rights offices investigating discrimination. Complaint processes vary by state.

Professional organizations: If provider is member of professional organization (American College of Obstetricians and Gynecologists, American Academy of Pediatrics, etc.), file complaints about ethics violations.

What to include in complaints:

- Your contact information
- Provider/institution names
- Specific dates and incidents
- Names of staff involved if known
- Description of discriminatory conduct
- How it harmed you or your family
- What resolution you're seeking
- Supporting documentation (emails, medical records, notes)

Potential outcomes: Complaints might result in policy changes, staff training, apologies, financial compensation, or disciplinary action against individual providers. Or they might result in nothing—bureaucracies protect themselves. File anyway. Patterns of complaints eventually force change.

30.3 Working with Patient Advocates

Patient advocates exist to mediate between patients and healthcare institutions, solving problems that frontline staff can't or won't address.

What patient advocates do:

- Investigate patient complaints
- Mediate conflicts between patients and providers
- Connect patients with resources
- Facilitate communication with medical teams
- Help navigate hospital systems
- Advocate for policy changes addressing repeated problems

How to access patient advocates: Most hospitals have patient advocacy offices or patient relations departments. Ask at hospital information desks, call the main hospital number, or check hospital websites. Some insurance companies also provide patient advocates.

What to bring to patient advocates:

- Documentation of problems (dates, incidents, people involved)
- Copies of relevant medical records or forms
- Clear description of what's happened
- Specific requests for resolution

Effective advocacy requests:

- "I need all hospital forms updated to include options for two mothers or two fathers, not just 'mother' and 'father.'"
- "Staff keep misgendering me despite corrections. I need mandatory training on transgender patient care and accountability for staff who refuse to use correct pronouns."
- "My partner has been excluded from medical discussions despite being a legal parent. I need explicit protocols ensuring both parents receive information."

Following up: After meeting with patient advocates, follow up in writing summarizing what was discussed and what actions were promised. Request confirmation in writing. Follow up again if promised changes don't happen.

Escalating beyond patient advocates: If patient advocates don't resolve issues, escalate to hospital administrators, file complaints with licensing agencies, or contact LGBTQ+ legal advocacy organizations for support.

30.4 Educating Providers in Real Time

Sometimes providers lack knowledge about LGBTQ+ families but are open to learning. Educational advocacy differs from combative advocacy—it assumes good intent and offers information.

When education works: With providers who make mistakes but respond positively to correction, who ask questions respectfully, or who acknowledge their lack of knowledge and want to improve.

When education doesn't work: With providers who are hostile, who refuse to acknowledge mistakes, or who repeatedly make the same errors despite education. These providers need complaints, not patient education.

How to educate effectively:

Provide written resources: Prepare one-page summaries about transgender pregnancy, family structures with two mothers or two fathers, or inclusive language. Hand these to providers who seem receptive. Organizations like GLMA (health professionals advancing LGBTQ+ equality) provide free downloadable resources.

Offer specific language: Instead of saying "don't misgender me," try "I prefer to use the term 'chest-feeding' instead of 'breastfeeding.' Can you make note of that in my chart?" Specific suggestions are easier to implement than vague requests.

Frame as professional development: "I know you might not have many LGBTQ+ patients, so I wanted to share some information that might help with future patients too." This positions you as collaborator rather than complainer.

Acknowledge improvement: When providers make efforts to improve, acknowledge it: "I noticed you used my correct pronouns throughout the appointment today. Thank you—that matters a lot." Positive reinforcement encourages continued effort.

Know when to stop: Don't exhaust yourself educating providers who aren't receptive. It's not your job to train medical professionals. Do what feels sustainable and stop when it's too much.

30.5 Sharing Your Story

Sharing your experience publicly—through social media, interviews, writing, or speaking—creates visibility and change. But sharing is optional and not without risk.

Benefits of sharing:

- Helps other LGBTQ+ people feel less alone
- Educates general public about LGBTQ+ family building
- Pressures institutions to change through public accountability
- Connects you with community
- Contributes to cultural shift toward acceptance

Risks of sharing:

- Invites judgment and criticism
- Exposes your family to public scrutiny
- Might affect employment or housing
- Opens door to harassment
- Reduces privacy

Deciding whether to share: Consider your specific circumstances—employment stability, geographic location, family relationships, mental health capacity, desire for privacy. Sharing isn't morally superior to staying private. Both choices are valid.

If you choose to share:

Control your narrative: Tell your story on your terms. You don't have to answer every invasive question. Set boundaries about what's private versus public.

Choose platforms carefully: Some platforms amplify voices better than others. Consider whether you want local impact (local news, community organizations) or broader reach (social media, national media, podcasts).

Protect children's privacy: Consider how sharing affects your children now and in the future. Many LGBTQ+ parents share their own stories while protecting children's identities.

Prepare for backlash: Visible LGBTQ+ people receive hate. Develop strategies for managing negative responses—moderating comments, blocking harassers, taking breaks from social media.

Connect with others sharing stories: Organizations like Family Equality coordinate storytelling campaigns and provide support for people sharing publicly.

30.6 Supporting Policy Change

Individual advocacy helps your family. Policy advocacy creates systemic change protecting all LGBTQ+ families.

Policy issues affecting LGBTQ+ families:

- Birth certificate laws recognizing both same-sex parents
- Second-parent adoption accessibility and affordability
- Insurance coverage for fertility treatments regardless of relationship status
- Anti-discrimination protections in healthcare
- Parental leave policies including non-gestational parents
- School policies recognizing diverse family structures

How to support policy change:

Contact legislators: Call, email, or visit your local, state, and federal legislators about LGBTQ+ family issues. Personal constituent stories are powerful—legislators listen more to constituents than to advocacy organizations.

Testify at hearings: Many legislative committees hold public hearings on proposed laws. Testifying puts human faces on policy issues.

Join advocacy organizations: Family Equality, COLAGE, National Center for Lesbian Rights, and other organizations coordinate policy advocacy. Joining amplifies your voice through collective action.

Support LGBTQ+ friendly candidates: Vote for candidates supporting LGBTQ+ rights. Donate to campaigns if possible. Volunteer on campaigns.

Participate in campaigns: Many policy changes result from organized campaigns—letter-writing campaigns, petition drives, coordinated call-in days. Participate when these opportunities arise.

Support local change: National policy matters, but local policies affect daily life. Advocate for LGBTQ+-inclusive policies in your school district, local hospitals, municipal governments, and community organizations.

30.7 Building LGBTQ+ Parent Community

Individual advocacy is exhausting. Community makes advocacy sustainable and effective.

Why community matters:

- Shared advocacy is more effective than individual efforts
- Community provides support during difficult advocacy battles
- Collective action creates pressure for change
- Community shares resources and information
- You're less isolated when facing discrimination

Finding LGBTQ+ parent community:

- Local LGBTQ+ parenting groups (search on Facebook, Meetup, or through local LGBTQ+ centers)
- Family Equality's national network
- Online forums and social media groups
- LGBTQ+ parenting conferences
- Rainbow families at childcare, schools, and activities
- Support groups through LGBTQ+ health centers

Building community: If your area lacks LGBTQ+ parent community, start one. Post in local LGBTQ+ Facebook groups or parent groups. Host informal meetups at parks or coffee shops. Even connecting with one or two other LGBTQ+ families reduces isolation.

Supporting each other: Community means sharing resources—provider recommendations, legal referrals, childcare, meal trains during postpartum, advocacy strategies. Build reciprocal support networks.

Mentoring: As experienced LGBTQ+ parents, mentor people newer to the journey. Share what you've learned. Offer encouragement. The LGBTQ+ parent community grows stronger through intergenerational support.

30.8 Real Advocacy Journey

Consider Aisha and Layla's experience (composite): After their hospital refused to list both mothers on their daughter's birth certificate, they didn't just hire an attorney for their own case—they organized.

Aisha connected with other same-sex couples who'd had babies at the same hospital. Five families reported identical problems. Together, they met with the hospital's patient advocate with documentation from all five families showing a pattern of discrimination.

The patient advocate initially defended hospital policy, citing "state law." Aisha responded: "State law requires you to list both spouses on birth certificates under *Pavan v. Smith*. Your policy violates federal constitutional law."

When the patient advocate still resisted, the five families filed formal complaints with the state department of health, the hospital licensing board, and the U.S. Department of Health and Human

Services Office for Civil Rights. They also contacted local media. The hospital suddenly became very interested in resolving the issue.

Within two months, the hospital changed its policy, updated all forms to include options for two mothers or two fathers, and trained staff on LGBTQ+ family recognition. All five families received corrected birth certificates.

But Aisha and Layla didn't stop there. They testified at state legislative hearings about birth certificate discrimination. They shared their story in local news, putting faces to abstract legal arguments. They joined Family Equality's advocacy network.

Two years later, their advocacy contributed to state law changes strengthening LGBTQ+ parent recognition. Their individual discrimination experience became systemic change protecting families who came after them.

30.9 Core Advocacy Principles

Self-advocacy means clearly stating your needs, correcting mistakes immediately, and escalating when necessary. File formal complaints when discrimination occurs—with hospital patient advocates, licensing boards, civil rights offices, and professional organizations. Document everything to support complaints.

Patient advocates mediate between patients and institutions, investigating complaints and facilitating resolution. Educate providers who are receptive, offering specific language and written resources, but don't exhaust yourself educating hostile providers. Sharing your story publicly creates visibility but involves risks—decide based on your circumstances.

Support policy change through contacting legislators, testifying at hearings, joining advocacy organizations, and participating in campaigns. Build LGBTQ+ parent community for mutual support and collective advocacy power. Individual advocacy protects your family; systemic advocacy creates lasting change benefiting all

LGBTQ+ families. You don't have to fight every battle, but the battles you choose to fight make the world safer for families who come after you.

Appendices

Appendix A: Provider Question Bank

Questions for Midwives

Initial Consultation:

- How many LGBTQ+ families have you served?
- How do you document two mothers, two fathers, or transgender parents?
- What's your experience with transgender pregnancy specifically?
- How do you handle pronouns and preferred terminology?
- Can my partner be fully involved in all appointments and birth?
- What's your philosophy on gender-neutral or inclusive language?

Clinical Care:

- How do you approach chest-feeding or breastfeeding support for transgender men?
- What's your experience managing dysphoria during pregnancy and postpartum?
- How do you ensure both parents receive postpartum care information?
- What resources do you provide for LGBTQ+ families specifically?

Birth Planning:

- How do you advocate for LGBTQ+ families in hospital settings?
- What happens if I face discrimination during labor?
- How do you ensure my partner has full access during birth?

- What's your backup plan if you're unavailable for birth?

Questions for OBs

Practice Policies:

- How many LGBTQ+ patients does your practice serve?
- What training has your staff received on LGBTQ+ care?
- How are intake forms structured—do they accommodate diverse families?
- How do you ensure all staff use correct names and pronouns?
- What's your practice's non-discrimination policy?

Pregnancy Care:

- How do you involve non-gestational partners in care?
- What's your experience with fertility treatment pregnancies?
- How do you approach prenatal testing and genetic counseling for donor-conceived pregnancies?
- What accommodations do you make for patients with dysphoria?

Birth and Postpartum:

- What hospital(s) do you deliver at, and how LGBTQ+-friendly are they?
- How do you handle birth certificate completion for same-sex parents?
- What postpartum support do you provide for both parents?
- How do you coordinate care between OB and pediatrician for our family?

Questions for Fertility Specialists

Practice Experience:

- What percentage of your patients are LGBTQ+ individuals or couples?
- Do you have experience with transgender men seeking fertility preservation or pregnancy?
- How do you approach fertility care for non-binary individuals?
- What's your success rate specifically with LGBTQ+ patients?

Treatment Options:

- What fertility treatment options do you recommend for our situation?
- How do you select sperm donors or egg donors?
- What's your clinic's policy on known donors versus anonymous donors?
- How do you handle legal agreements for known donors?
- What are realistic success rates and timelines for our specific situation?

Costs and Insurance:

- What are total costs for each treatment option?
- What does insurance cover and what's out-of-pocket?
- Do you offer payment plans or financing?
- Are there less expensive options we should consider first?

Emotional Support:

- What mental health support do you provide during fertility treatment?
- How do you support couples through fertility treatment stress?
- What resources exist for LGBTQ+ people specifically going through fertility treatment?

Questions for Pediatricians

Practice Philosophy:

- How many LGBTQ+ families do you serve?
- How do you document multiple mothers, multiple fathers, or transgender parents in your system?
- What training has your staff received on diverse family structures?
- How do you ensure respectful care for all family types?

Care Approach:

- How do you involve both parents in medical decisions?
- What's your communication approach—do both parents receive test results and medical information?
- How do you handle situations where only one parent is legally recognized?
- What's your approach to discussing our family structure with our child as they grow?

Practical Matters:

- What are your office hours and availability for sick visits?
- How do you handle after-hours calls or emergencies?
- What hospital are you affiliated with?
- What's your vaccine philosophy?
- How do you approach common controversial topics (circumcision, sleep training, etc.)?

Questions for Mental Health Providers

Experience and Training:

- What's your experience working with LGBTQ+ individuals and couples?
- Do you have specific training in perinatal mental health?
- What's your experience with gender dysphoria during pregnancy and postpartum?

- Are you familiar with minority stress and its impact on LGBTQ+ people?

Treatment Approach:

- What's your therapeutic orientation or approach?
- How do you address both individual and relationship issues?
- What's your experience treating postpartum depression and anxiety?
- How do you approach trauma related to discrimination or past negative healthcare experiences?

Practical Information:

- What insurance do you accept?
- What are your fees if paying out-of-pocket?
- What's your availability for appointments?
- Do you offer telehealth options?
- Can you see both partners individually and as a couple?

Appendix B: Document Templates

Birth Preferences Template

Our Family:

- Birthing person's name and pronouns:
- Partner's name and pronouns:
- Preferred terminology (pregnant person/mother/father/parent/chest-feeding/breastfeeding):

Labor Preferences:

- Pain management preferences:
- Movement and positioning freedom:
- Who we want present:
- Things to avoid:

Birth Preferences:

- Pushing positions:
- Assisted delivery if needed:
- Cesarean preferences if necessary:
- Delayed cord clamping: Yes/No
- Skin-to-skin immediately after birth: Yes/No

Newborn Care:

- Vitamin K injection: Yes/No
- Eye ointment: Yes/No
- Hepatitis B vaccine: Yes/No
- Circumcision (if applicable): Yes/No
- Feeding plan:
- Rooming in versus nursery:

Important for Our Family:

- Both parents must be included in all decisions and information
- Use our correct names and pronouns consistently
- Respect our privacy and family structure
- Birth certificate must list both parents correctly

Hospital Communication Letter

To Hospital Staff:

We are expecting our baby on [date] at [hospital name]. We want to ensure respectful, inclusive care for our family.

Our Family Structure: [Describe your family—e.g., "We are two mothers," "I am a transgender man and my wife is my partner," etc.]

Essential Information:

- Birthing person's name, pronouns, and preferred terms:
- Partner's name, pronouns, and role:
- Both parents have legal parental rights: [Yes/No—if no, explain]
- Partner must be included in all medical discussions and decisions
- Partner must have 24/7 access to birthing person

Specific Requests:

- Use our correct names and pronouns consistently
- Update all forms and systems to reflect our family structure
- Include both parents on birth certificate paperwork
- Provide lactation support using our preferred terminology
- Respect our privacy—don't share details about our family structure with staff who don't need to know

Contact Information: If questions arise about our care or family structure, please contact:

- Our OB/midwife: [name and phone]
- Patient advocate: [name and phone]
- Our attorney (if applicable): [name and phone]

We expect professional, respectful care. Thank you for supporting our family.

Sincerely, [Names and signatures]

Partner Agreement Template

Co-Parenting Agreement Between [Name] and [Name]

This agreement, made on [date], establishes our intentions regarding the conception, birth, and parenting of our child(ren).

Our Intentions: We intend to conceive and raise a child together as equal co-parents with shared custody, decision-making authority, and financial responsibility.

Conception Method: We plan to conceive using [IUI/IVF/home insemination/other] with [sperm donor/egg donor/gestational carrier].

Parental Rights:

- Both parties will be legal parents with equal rights and responsibilities
- [Non-biological parent] will complete second-parent adoption if required
- Both parties will be listed on birth certificate
- Both parties will have medical decision-making authority

Financial Responsibilities:

- Pregnancy and birth costs will be shared: [specify arrangement]
- Childcare costs will be shared: [specify arrangement]

- Child support: [specify arrangement if relationship ends]

Living Arrangements: We intend to [live together/co-parent from separate households/other arrangement].

If Relationship Ends:

- Custody arrangement: [specify intended arrangement]
- Child support obligations: [specify arrangement]
- Decision-making: [specify arrangement]

Dispute Resolution: If disputes arise, we agree to attempt mediation before pursuing litigation.

Legal Effect: This agreement represents our intentions and may be used as evidence of parental intent, though it may not be legally binding depending on jurisdiction. We understand we may need formal legal agreements (second-parent adoption, custody agreements) to ensure enforceability.

Signatures: ______________________________ Date: ____________ [Name]

______________________________ Date: ____________ [Name]

Note: This template is for planning purposes. Consult with an attorney to create a legally binding agreement.

Known Donor Agreement Template

Sperm Donation Agreement Between [Donor Name] and [Recipient Name(s)]

This agreement, made on [date], establishes the understanding between sperm donor and recipient(s) regarding donation and parental rights.

Parties:

- Donor: [Name, address]
- Recipient(s): [Name(s), address(es)]

Intentions:

- Donor agrees to provide sperm for the purpose of conception
- Recipient(s) intend to conceive and parent the resulting child(ren)
- Donor [does/does not] intend to have ongoing relationship with child

Parental Rights and Obligations:

- Donor waives all parental rights and has no custody, visitation, or decision-making rights
- Donor has no financial obligations (child support) for resulting child(ren)
- Recipient(s) will be sole legal parent(s) with full parental rights
- Recipient(s) assume all financial responsibility for child(ren)

Contact with Child:

- Donor [will/will not] have ongoing contact with child
- If contact: [specify nature and frequency]
- Child [will/will not] know donor's identity

Medical Information:

- Donor provides complete medical history (attached)
- Donor agrees to update recipients if significant medical conditions develop
- Donor agrees to STI testing before donation

Confidentiality:

- Parties agree to [maintain confidentiality/allow information sharing/other]

Compensation:

- Donor [is/is not] being compensated
- If compensated: [specify amount and terms]

Legal Understanding: We understand that this agreement may or may not be legally enforceable depending on jurisdiction and specific circumstances. We understand that legal parentage is determined by state law and that this agreement cannot override state law regarding parental rights. We strongly recommend both parties consult with attorneys familiar with reproductive law in our state.

Signatures: ______________________________ Date: ____________ [Donor name]

______________________________ Date: ____________ [Recipient name]

______________________________ Date: ____________ [Recipient name, if applicable]

Note: This template is not a substitute for legal advice. Consult with a reproductive law attorney in your state before entering into a known donor arrangement.

Healthcare Proxy Form

[Your State] Healthcare Proxy

I, ____________________________ (your name), residing at ____________________________ (address), appoint:

____________________________ (agent's name)
____________________________ (agent's address)
____________________________ (agent's phone)

as my healthcare agent to make healthcare decisions for me if I become unable to make them myself.

Agent's Authority: My agent has authority to:

- Consent to, refuse, or withdraw any medical treatment or procedure
- Access my medical records
- Make decisions about life-sustaining treatment
- Make decisions about organ donation
- Authorize hospitalization or placement in care facilities

Specific Instructions: [Include any specific instructions about life-sustaining treatment, organ donation, or other healthcare preferences]

Alternate Agent: If my first agent is unavailable, I appoint: ___________________________ (alternate agent's name and contact information)

Effective Date: This proxy becomes effective when: [my physician determines I lack capacity/immediately upon signing/other]

Duration: This proxy remains in effect unless I revoke it.

Signature: ______________________________ Date: ____________ [Your signature]

Witnesses: ______________________________ Date: ____________ [Witness 1 signature, name, address]

______________________________ Date: ____________ [Witness 2 signature, name, address]

Note: Healthcare proxy requirements vary by state. Consult your state's specific forms and requirements.

Appendix C: Resource Directory

National LGBTQ+ Organizations

Family Equality www.familyequality.org National advocacy organization supporting LGBTQ+ families through community building, advocacy, and resources.

COLAGE (Children of Lesbians and Gays Everywhere) www.colage.org Organization supporting people with LGBTQ+ parents through community, advocacy, and resources.

National Center for Lesbian Rights (NCLR) www.nclrights.org Legal organization providing free and low-cost legal services to LGBTQ+ people and families.

Lambda Legal www.lambdalegal.org National legal organization fighting for LGBTQ+ rights through litigation and advocacy.

GLMA: Health Professionals Advancing LGBTQ+ Equality www.glma.org Organization of LGBTQ+ healthcare professionals promoting inclusive healthcare.

Transgender Law Center www.transgenderlawcenter.org Legal organization supporting transgender people through legal services and advocacy.

Human Rights Campaign (HRC) www.hrc.org National LGBTQ+ advocacy organization with resources on family building and parenting.

Fertility and Family Building Resources

Path2Parenthood www.path2parenthood.org Organization supporting people facing fertility challenges, including LGBTQ+ specific resources.

RESOLVE: The National Infertility Association www.resolve.org Provides fertility information and support with resources for LGBTQ+ family building.

Men Having Babies www.menhavingbabies.org Organization supporting gay men pursuing surrogacy and adoption.

Gay Parents To Be www.gayparentstobe.com Resource directory for LGBTQ+ family building options and support.

Mental Health Support

Postpartum Support International www.postpartum.net 1-800-944-4773 Organization providing support for perinatal mental health conditions, including LGBTQ+ resources.

Trevor Project www.thetrevorproject.org 1-866-488-7386 Crisis support for LGBTQ+ youth (useful for LGBTQ+ parents experiencing crisis).

Trans Lifeline www.translifeline.org 1-877-565-8860 Crisis hotline and support services for transgender people.

NAMI (National Alliance on Mental Illness) www.nami.org Mental health organization with resources and support groups nationwide.

Legal Resources

National Center for Lesbian Rights (NCLR) Legal Help www.nclrights.org/get-help Free legal consultations for LGBTQ+ people facing legal issues.

Lambda Legal Help Desk www.lambdalegal.org/help Free legal advice for LGBTQ+ people nationwide.

American Civil Liberties Union (ACLU) LGBTQ+ Rights Project www.aclu.org/issues/lgbtq-rights Legal support and resources for LGBTQ+ rights violations.

Transgender Legal Defense & Education Fund www.transgenderlegal.org Legal services for transgender people facing discrimination.

Pregnancy Loss Support

The Compassionate Friends www.compassionatefriends.org Support for families after death of a child, including pregnancy loss.

Return to Zero: H.O.P.E. www.rtzhope.org Support and resources for pregnancy loss and infant loss.

Star Legacy Foundation www.starlegacyfoundation.org Support for stillbirth and pregnancy loss with family-centered resources.

Finding LGBTQ+ Affirming Providers

GLMA Provider Directory www.glma.org/provider-directory Directory of LGBTQ+-affirming healthcare providers nationwide.

OutCare www.outcarehealth.org Searchable database of LGBTQ+ competent healthcare providers.

RAD Remedy www.radremedy.org Community-driven database of LGBTQ+-friendly healthcare providers.

Psychology Today Therapist Finder www.psychologytoday.com/us/therapists Search for therapists specializing in LGBTQ+ issues and perinatal mental health.

State-Specific Legal Information

Movement Advancement Project (MAP) www.lgbtmap.org State-by-state information on LGBTQ+ laws and policies, including parental recognition laws.

National Center for Lesbian Rights State-by-State Guide www.nclrights.org/our-work/policy/state-by-state Information on second-parent adoption and parental rights laws by state.

Financial Assistance and Grants

Family Equality LGBTQ Family Building Survey www.familyequality.org Periodic grants and financial assistance for LGBTQ+ family building.

Men Having Babies Surrogacy Financing www.menhavingbabies.org/financial-assistance Financial assistance programs for gay men pursuing surrogacy.

Cade Foundation www.cadefoundation.org Grants for LGBTQ+ individuals pursuing family building.

Appendix D: Evidence-Based Reference Guide

Key Studies on LGBTQ+ Perinatal Health

Transgender Pregnancy: Light, A. D., Obedin-Maliver, J., Sevelius, J. M., & Kerns, J. L. (2014). Transgender men who experienced pregnancy after female-to-male gender transitioning. *Obstetrics & Gynecology, 124*(6), 1120-1127.

Same-Sex Parent Outcomes: Gartrell, N. K., Bos, H. M., & Koh, A. S. (2018). National Longitudinal Lesbian Family Study—Mental health of adult offspring. *New England Journal of Medicine, 379*(3), 297-299.

Minority Stress in LGBTQ+ Pregnancy: Bos, H. M., & van Balen, F. (2010). Children of the new reproductive technologies: Social and genetic parenthood. *Patient Education and Counseling, 81*(3), 429-435.

Lactation in Transgender Men: MacDonald, T., Noel-Weiss, J., West, D., Walks, M., Biener, M., Kibbe, A., & Myler, E. (2016). Transmasculine individuals' experiences with lactation, chestfeeding, and gender identity: A qualitative study. *BMC Pregnancy and Childbirth, 16*(1), 106.

Clinical Guidelines and Position Statements

American College of Obstetricians and Gynecologists (ACOG):

- Committee Opinion No. 512: Healthcare for transgender individuals (2021)
- Committee Opinion No. 731: Group prenatal care (2018)

World Professional Association for Transgender Health (WPATH):

- Standards of Care for the Health of Transsexual, Transgender, and Gender Nonconforming People, Version 8 (2022)

American Academy of Pediatrics:

- Policy Statement: Ensuring comprehensive care and support for transgender and gender-diverse children and adolescents (2018)

Medication Safety Resources

LactMed (Drugs and Lactation Database) National Library of Medicine www.ncbi.nlm.nih.gov/books/NBK501922 Evidence-based information on medication safety during lactation.

MotherToBaby Organization of Teratology Information Specialists (OTIS) www.mothertobaby.org Free counseling on medication safety during pregnancy and breastfeeding.

Infant Risk Center Hotline Texas Tech University Health Sciences Center 1-806-352-2519 Pharmacist-staffed hotline providing medication safety information for pregnant and lactating people.

Clinical Practice Resources for Providers

GLMA Guidelines for Care of Lesbian, Gay, Bisexual, and Transgender Patients
www.glma.org/_data/n_0001/resources/live/GLMA%20guidelines%202006%20FINAL.pdf

Fenway Health's National LGBT Health Education Center
www.lgbtqiahealtheducation.org Free continuing medical education on LGBTQ+ health topics.

Center of Excellence for Transgender Health, UCSF
www.transhealth.ucsf.edu Clinical guidelines for transgender health care.

Human Rights Campaign Healthcare Equality Index
www.hrc.org/hei Annual rating of healthcare facilities on LGBTQ+ inclusion.

Organization

By Chapter: References are organized by chapter, allowing readers to find research supporting specific topics.

Format: All references follow APA 7th edition format with DOIs or stable URLs when available.

Categories:

- Peer-reviewed research from PubMed and academic databases
- Clinical guidelines from professional organizations
- Government reports and statistics
- Community resources and advocacy publications

References

- **American Academy of Pediatrics Task Force on Circumcision. (2012).** Male circumcision. *Pediatrics, 130*(3), e756–e785.
- **American College of Obstetricians and Gynecologists. (2018).** Early pregnancy loss. *ACOG Practice Bulletin No. 200.*
- **American College of Obstetricians and Gynecologists. (2018).** Gestational diabetes mellitus. *ACOG Practice Bulletin No. 190.*
- **American College of Obstetricians and Gynecologists. (2020).** Gestational hypertension and preeclampsia. *ACOG Practice Bulletin No. 222.*
- **American College of Obstetricians and Gynecologists. (2021).** Postpartum depression. (FAQ).
- **American College of Obstetricians and Gynecologists. (2023).** Morning sickness: Nausea and vomiting of pregnancy. (FAQ).
- **American College of Obstetricians and Gynecologists. (2023).** Preeclampsia and high blood pressure during pregnancy. (FAQ).
- **American Diabetes Association. (2023).** Management of diabetes in pregnancy: Standards of care in diabetes. *Diabetes Care, 46*(Suppl. 1), S254–S266.
- **American Society for Reproductive Medicine. (2012).** Age and fertility: A guide for patients. *Fertility and Sterility, 98*(5), 1125–1127.
- **American Society for Reproductive Medicine. (2021).** Access to fertility treatment irrespective of marital status, sexual orientation, or gender identity: An Ethics Committee opinion. *Fertility and Sterility.*
- **American Society for Reproductive Medicine. (2023).** Infertility: An overview.
- **Al-Kuran, O., Al-Mehaisen, L., Bawadi, H., Beitawi, S., & Amarin, Z. (2011).** The effect of late pregnancy

consumption of date fruit on labour and delivery. *Journal of Obstetrics and Gynaecology, 31*(1), 29–31.

- **Albers, L. L. (1999).** The duration of labor in healthy women. *Journal of Perinatology, 19*(2), 114–119.
- **Ayers, S., Bond, R., Bertullies, S., & Wijma, K. (2016).** The aetiology of post-traumatic stress following childbirth: A meta-analysis and theoretical framework. *Psychological Medicine, 46*(6), 1121–1134.
- **Azziz, R., Carmina, E., Chen, Z., Dunaif, A., Laven, J. S., Legro, R. S., … Yildiz, B. O. (2016).** Polycystic ovary syndrome. *Nature Reviews Disease Primers, 2*, 16057.
- **Beckmann, M. M., & Stock, O. M. (2013).** Antenatal perineal massage for reducing perineal trauma. *Cochrane Database of Systematic Reviews, 4*, CD005123.
- **Begley, C. M., Gyte, G. M., Devane, D., McGuire, W., Weeks, A., & Biesty, L. M. (2019).** Active versus expectant management for the third stage of labour. *Cochrane Database of Systematic Reviews, 2*, CD007412.
- **Bohren, M. A., Hofmeyr, G. J., Sakala, C., Fukuzawa, R. K., & Cuthbert, A. (2017).** Continuous support for women during childbirth. *Cochrane Database of Systematic Reviews, 7*, CD003766.
- **Bostock v. Clayton County, 590 U.S. 644 (2020).**
- **Cahill, S. R., Singal, R., Grasso, C., King, D., Mayer, K., Baker, K., & Makadon, H. J. (2014).** Do ask, do tell: Acceptability of routine collection of sexual orientation and gender identity data. *PLOS ONE, 9*(9), e107104.
- **Caplan, A. L., & Levine, A. D. (2017).** Hope, hype, and help: Ethically assessing the growing market in stem cell treatments. *The American Journal of Bioethics, 17*(5), 24–25.
- **Cassidy, P. R. (2018).** Care quality following intrauterine death in Spanish hospitals: Results from an online survey. *BMC Pregnancy and Childbirth, 18*, 22.
- **Chabot, J. M., & Ames, B. D. (2004).** "It wasn't 'let's get pregnant and go do it'": Decision making in lesbian couples planning motherhood via donor insemination. *Family Relations, 53*(4), 348–356.

- **Dennis, C.-L., Falah-Hassani, K., & Shiri, R. (2017).** Prevalence of antenatal and postnatal anxiety: Systematic review and meta-analysis. *British Journal of Psychiatry, 210*(5), 315–323.
- **Dempsey, D. (2013).** Surrogacy, gay male couples and the significance of biogenetic paternity. *New Genetics and Society, 32*(1), 37–53.
- **Doss, B. D., Rhoades, G. K., Stanley, S. M., & Markman, H. J. (2009).** The effect of the transition to parenthood on relationship quality: An 8-year prospective study. *Journal of Personality and Social Psychology, 96*(3), 601–619.
- **Ethics Committee of the American Society for Reproductive Medicine. (2013).** Access to fertility treatment by gays, lesbians, and unmarried persons: A committee opinion. *Fertility and Sterility, 100*(6), 1524–1527.
- **Fairbrother, N., Janssen, P., Antony, M. M., Tucker, E., & Young, A. H. (2016).** Perinatal anxiety disorder prevalence and incidence. *Journal of Affective Disorders, 200*, 148–155.
- **Family Equality. (2019).** LGBTQ Family Building Survey.
- **Family Equality. (2023).** Family building financial assistance.
- **Ferrara, I., Balet, R., & Grudzinskas, J. G. (2018).** Intrauterine insemination with frozen donor sperm. *Reproductive BioMedicine Online, 36*(6), 656–666.
- **Fillo, J., Alfano, L., Payne, E., & Kiel, E. J. (2015).** Partner effects on early parenting stress: Relation to maternal and paternal depression and anxiety. *Archives of Women's Mental Health, 18*(2), 287–295.
- **Gadsby, R., Barnie-Adshead, A. M., & Jagger, C. (1993).** A prospective study of nausea and vomiting during pregnancy. *British Journal of General Practice, 43*(371), 245–248.
- **Goldfarb, L., & Newman, J. (2019).** *The Newman–Goldfarb protocols for induced lactation: A guide for maximizing breastmilk production.* AskLenore.

- **Giudice, L. C. (2010).** Clinical practice: Endometriosis. *New England Journal of Medicine, 362*(25), 2389–2398.
- **GLMA: Health Professionals Advancing LGBTQ Equality. (2023).** Provider directory.
- **Goldberg, A. E. (2006).** The transition to parenthood for lesbian couples. *Journal of GLBT Family Studies, 2*(1), 13–42.
- **Goldberg, A. E., & Perry-Jenkins, M. (2007).** The division of labor and perceptions of parental roles: Lesbian couples across the transition to parenthood. *Journal of Social and Personal Relationships, 24*(2), 297–318.
- **Goodman, J. H., Watson, G. R., & Stubbs, B. (2016).** Anxiety disorders in postpartum women: A systematic review and meta-analysis. *Journal of Affective Disorders, 203*, 292–331.
- **Grobman, W. A., Rice, M. M., Reddy, U. M., Tita, A. T. N., Silver, R. M., … NICHD MFMU Network. (2018).** Labor induction versus expectant management in low-risk nulliparous women. *New England Journal of Medicine, 379*(6), 513–523.
- **Grummer-Strawn, L. M., & Rollins, N. (2015).** Summarising the health effects of breastfeeding. *Acta Paediatrica, 104*(S467), 1–2.
- **Hoffkling, A., Obedin-Maliver, J., & Sevelius, J. (2017).** From erasure to opportunity: Experiences of transgender men around pregnancy. *BMC Pregnancy and Childbirth, 17*(Suppl 2), 332.
- **Human Milk Banking Association of North America. (2023).** About donor milk.
- **Institute of Medicine. (2009).** *Weight gain during pregnancy: Reexamining the guidelines.* National Academies Press.
- **Lambda Legal. (2010).** When health care isn't caring: Survey of discrimination against LGBT people and people with HIV.
- **Lambda Legal. (2020).** Know your rights: Healthcare.
- **Light, A. D., Obedin-Maliver, J., Sevelius, J. M., & Kerns, J. L. (2014).** Transgender men who experienced

pregnancy after female-to-male gender transitioning. *Obstetrics & Gynecology, 124*(6), 1120–1127.

- **Louis, G. M., Lum, K. J., Sundaram, R., Chen, Z., Kim, S., Lynch, C. D., … Pyper, C. (2011).** Stress reduces conception probabilities across the fertile window. *Fertility and Sterility, 95*(7), 2184–2189.
- **March of Dimes. (2021).** The cost of having a baby in the United States.
- **March of Dimes. (2023).** Premature birth report card.
- **Martin, J. A., Hamilton, B. E., & Osterman, M. J. K. (2021).** Births: Final data for 2020. *National Vital Statistics Reports, 70*(17).
- **Matorras, R., Prieto, B., Exposito, A., Mendoza, R., Crisol, L., Herranz, P., & Burgues, S. (2015).** Mid-follicular LH supplementation in women aged 35–39 years undergoing ICSI. *Reproductive BioMedicine Online, 30*(2), 179–187.
- **McDonald, S. J., Middleton, P., Dowswell, T., & Morris, P. S. (2013).** Timing of umbilical cord clamping at term. *Cochrane Database of Systematic Reviews, 7*, CD004074.
- **Moon, R. Y., & Task Force on Sudden Infant Death Syndrome. (2016).** SIDS and other sleep-related infant deaths: 2016 recommendations. *Pediatrics, 138*(5), e20162938.
- **Moore, E. R., Bergman, N., Anderson, G. C., & Medley, N. (2016).** Early skin-to-skin contact for mothers and healthy newborns. *Cochrane Database of Systematic Reviews, 11*, CD003519.
- **National Center for Lesbian Rights. (2022).** LGBT families and relationships: Know your rights.
- **National Center for Transgender Equality. (2021).** Know your rights: Healthcare.
- **Obedin-Maliver, J., & Makadon, H. J. (2016).** Transgender men and pregnancy. *Obstetric Medicine, 9*(1), 4–8.
- **Paulson, J. F., & Bazemore, S. D. (2010).** Prenatal and postpartum depression in fathers and association with maternal depression. *JAMA, 303*(19), 1961–1969.

- **Perritt, J. B. (2017).** LGBT inclusion: Legal and regulatory frameworks in reproductive health. *Seminars in Reproductive Medicine, 35*(4), 311–318.
- **Prins, M., Boxem, J., Lucas, C., & Hutton, E. (2011).** Spontaneous versus Valsalva pushing in the second stage: Systematic review. *BJOG, 118*(6), 662–670.
- **Ross, L. E., Steele, L., & Epstein, R. (2006).** Lesbian and bisexual women's experiences of maternity care in Toronto. *Canadian Journal of Midwifery Research and Practice, 5*(1), 8–15.
- **Sandall, J., Soltani, H., Gates, S., Shennan, A., & Devane, D. (2016).** Midwife-led continuity models versus other models of care. *Cochrane Database of Systematic Reviews, 4*, CD004667.
- **Society for Assisted Reproductive Technology. (2022).** National summary report.
- **Shorey, S., He, H. G., & Morelius, E. (2016).** Skin-to-skin contact by fathers: An integrative review. *Midwifery, 40*, 207–217.
- **Sockol, L. E. (2015).** Efficacy of cognitive behavioral therapy for perinatal depression: Systematic review. *Journal of Affective Disorders, 177*, 7–21.
- **Stapleton, L. R., Schetter, C. D., Westling, E., Rini, C., Glynn, L. M., Hobel, C. J., & Sandman, C. A. (2012).** Perceived partner support in pregnancy predicts lower maternal and infant distress. *Journal of Family Psychology, 26*(3), 453–463.
- **U.S. Equal Employment Opportunity Commission. (2023).** Pregnancy discrimination.
- **VanderKruik, R., Barreix, M., Chou, D., Allen, T., Say, L., & Cohen, L. S. (2017).** Global prevalence of postpartum psychosis: Systematic review. *BMC Psychiatry, 17*, 272.
- **Wilcox, A. J., Weinberg, C. R., & Baird, D. D. (1995).** Timing of intercourse in relation to ovulation and probability of conception. *New England Journal of Medicine, 333*(23), 1517–1521.
- **Wong, L. F., Schliep, K. C., Silver, R. M., Mumford, S. L., Perkins, N. J., Ye, A., … Schisterman, E. F. (2015).**

The effect of a very short interpregnancy interval after a prior pregnancy loss. *American Journal of Obstetrics and Gynecology, 212*(3), 375.e1–375.e11.

- **World Professional Association for Transgender Health. (2023).** Provider directory.

Made in the USA
Monee, IL
04 November 2026

67386636R00216